IN DEFENSE
OF THE BODY

23-28
34-38

7-13

IN DEFENSE OF THE BODY

An Introduction to
the New Immunology

ROGER LEWIN

Anchor Books
Anchor Press / Doubleday
Garden City, New York
1974

Anchor Books Edition: 1974
ISBN: 0-385-00379-X
Library of Congress Catalog Card Number 74-4900
Copyright © 1974 by Roger Lewin
Printed in the United States of America
First Edition

For

MARY, ADAM and JONATHAN

ACKNOWLEDGMENTS:

My thanks, as always, go to Mary, who this time was giving birth to a baby (Jonathan) as I was giving birth to this book. In spite of her substantial preoccupation Mary was always an inspiring source of encouragement and suggestions. During the past year I have talked to scores of research immunologists, and I am forever in their debt; particularly, my thanks to Tony Allison, Robert Good, Mel Greaves, John Humphrey, George Mathe, Avrion Mitchison and Ivan Roitt. I am deeply indebted to Professor Leslie Brent, who read through my manuscript and made many helpful comments. The responsibility for the final version is of course mine. Last, my thanks to Katherine Adams, whose typing speed never ceases to amaze me.

Contents

Contents

Introduction

The time is 1968; summer. Four young sisters are travelling with their parents from Connecticut to the University of Minnesota. The reason for the mass pilgrimage is their little brother, four months old, who seems doomed to die very young, just as eleven other boys in his family have over three generations. The boy, David Camp, is totally unable to defend himself from attack by bacteria, viruses and fungi. He is defenseless because he lacks a normal immune system. Immunology, the study of the body's immune mechanisms, is all about "self" and its defense against foreignness.

A few months after he arrived in Minnesota the death sentence had been lifted from David. One of his sisters donated some bone marrow—the seat of the immune system —which surgeons implanted into the boy's frail body. After a few disturbing complications the implanted bone marrow cells took up permanent residence in the boy's body and started performing the normal defensive role of the immune system. The man who inspired the pioneering bone marrow swap, Dr. Robert Good, now describes the whole incident as being "just like creating life." For David, his young life was snatched from an inexorable slide into a tragic death; for the doctors, a new approach had saved the first of many lives; and for immunology, a major milestone had been passed along the long, tortuous and exciting road to a complete understanding of the system.

Not that any scientist, even in a moment of manic hyperbole, would claim that immunologists can now pack up and go home because all the problems are solved. Far from it.

But the current explosion in immunological research throws out waves of discoveries that are giving insights into the science undreamed of a few years ago. Immunology is now one of the most rewarding and promising areas of biological research. It is rewarding because it spreads into many areas of acute social misery giving prospects of long-hoped-for cures: the successes of vaccinations against many bacterial and viral infections may soon be followed by assaults on cancer and diseases such a rheumatoid arthritis and the presently unassailable parasitic infections; immunology also holds the key to safe organ transplantations. And it is promising because the drive toward understanding the molecular mechanisms behind the immune responses is certain to reveal features fundamental to the whole of biology.

The Birth of Immunology

Immunology has not always been so sophisticated. The ancient Greeks knew about it. At least they knew that people who survived an attack of the plague were forever safe from the dreaded affliction—they were immune. The immunological defenses of the body "remember" that they have been challenged before by the plague, and they know how to combat it rapidly a second time. This phenomenon of "memory" is one of three key factors in the immune response.

However, should a survivor of the plague in ancient Greece —or modern America—come into contact with, say, smallpox, he will be just as vulnerable as anyone else. The immunological memory acquired by exposure to one disease is specific to that infection only. Although a person can become immune to a whole series of infections, the memory behind each immunity is specific for a particular foreign invader, whether it is smallpox virus or the tuberculosis bacterium. Specificity is the second major feature of the immune system. The remarkable degree of specificity displayed is rooted in intricate and fascinating molecular recognition mechanisms, as we shall see later.

Sometimes, however, this specificity falls short of complete: just as two people can look alike, so too can two viruses, at least to the immune defenses. It was the apparent similarity between the smallpox and cowpox viruses that set immunology toward its first golden era at the end of the eighteenth century. A young, clear-skinned milkmaid pointed out to Edward Jenner, a village doctor in rural England, that people who caught cowpox, as most milkmaids inevitably did, never succumbed to the dreaded smallpox (hence the absence of pockmarks on the milkmaid's skin).

Jenner was impressed by this astute observation and, in exploiting it, launched the now common clinical procedure —vaccination—which takes its name from that of the cowpox organism, vaccinia. He deliberately gave a young boy, James Phipps, a mild dose of cowpox; a few weeks later he took puss from smallpox sores and scratched it into Phipps's arm to see if the boy would succumb: he didn't. The immune defenses provoked by the cowpox viruses were also effective against the smallpox organisms. That was in 1798, long before anyone knew about the existence of bacteria, let alone viruses. Vaccination really took off, thus establishing immunology as a part of practical medicine, after the germ theory of disease emerged in the late 1800s. Only then did people have some idea what they were vaccinating against.

By 1950, when vaccines were available against a whole range of previously uncontrollable diseases, the boom in immunology seemed to be peaking out; the golden era was losing its glitter. Moreover, the appearance of the "magic" antibiotics which combated many infections, some of which immunology had failed to conquer, threatened to shift immunology into a historical perspective. But that was before the impact of the thrilling discoveries made by the molecular biologists in the 1960s.

The New Immunology

Molecular biology took life down to its finest detail, down to the shape and structure of the minute but enormously complex molecules that make us what we are. It showed how life's messages are carefully stored away in the genetic code, and how these messages are expressed in the form of the vitally important protein molecules. For immunology, it provided the means to examine how the body's cells interact, how they recognize each other as being "self" or "non-self." Because the immune response depends critically on the ability to recognize foreigners—the third major feature of the system—molecular biology helped generate a new and exciting era of immunology: molecular immunology.

Immunologists no longer look at a whole virus, say, as a potential invoker of an immune response. They want to know exactly which part of the virus is responsible, which molecule, which part of the molecule? And is it possible to fool the immune defenses by making an "artificial virus," a structure that carries only the immunologically important components? Scientists are now contemplating manipulating the immune system in a way that was inconceivable just a short time ago. This approach could be enormously important in the battle against cancer (which is a foreigner invading from within), because cancer escapes the normally vigilant attentions of the immune armory. Boosting the body's natural defenses to seek out and destroy normally recalcitrant tumors, and even vaccinating against cancer, are both very possible fruits of molecular immunology, better called the new immunology.

In this book we shall explore the secrets of the immune system's success: its *memory,* its *specificity* and its ability to *recognize foreignness.* We shall also try to understand its failures: in being not aggressive enough against cancer; being too aggressive both in the unfortunate cases of autoimmune diseases in which the system mistakes self for non-self, and in making life awkward for the transplant surgeon; and in being occasionally defective, thus causing immunodeficiency diseases.

Immunology is so all-pervading that it leaves no medical topic untouched. No wonder then that the new immunology is such an exciting story, a story moving so fast that it is almost impossible to keep pace with what is happening. The one certain thing about it is that for scientists, as for the public, immunology is very important, and will be increasingly so as each month passes.

1. Architecture of the Immune System

Specificity, memory and the ability to recognize foreignness are the key characteristics of the immune defense mechanisms. Our body's defenses must be able to recognize foreign invaders, such as bacteria and viruses, so that they can be tracked down and destroyed to prevent them colonizing our tissues and harming us. The defenses' specificity means that the search-and-destroy operations are maximally efficient. The memory facility allows a second challenge by an invader to be thrown off very rapidly. These three vital properties are invested in a single type of cell—the lymphocyte—which is one of the kinds of white cells that circulate in the blood.

It is symptomatic of the pace of recent research that lymphocytes, which now dominate the center of the immunological stage, were thought unworthy of a minor supporting role less than two decades ago. In the early 1960s James Gowans and Douglas McGregor of Oxford University finally proved the involvement of lymphocytes in the immune response. Now scientists know that these unpretentious little cells mediate the powerful response provoked by infection, that they elaborate intricate and sophisticated interrelationships between themselves. Most important, lymphocytes represent the prime target in scientists' attempts to manipulate the immune response.

The Components of the System

At any time there are a trillion lymphocytes in the human body which, in total, weigh two pounds. This is not a static

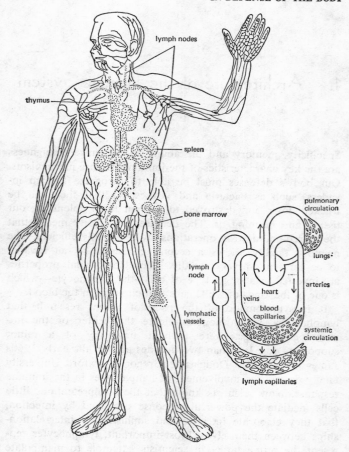

Figure 1. THE OVER-ALL STRUCTURE OF THE IMMUNE SYSTEM: Lymphocytes (white blood cells) and antibodies pass from the blood, through the body's tissues and into the lymphatic vessels. The lymphocytes are produced by the bone marrow and are processed either by the thymus gland or the spleen. The swellings scattered along the lymph vessels are known as lymph nodes; they contain many lymphocytes.

population: old ones are eliminated and new ones manufactured at a rate of almost 200,000 per second. The principal role of at least some of the lymphocytes is to manufacture and release special protein molecules, called antibodies, which represent part of the weaponry in the immunological armory. Every second of the day 20 trillion antibody molecules are spilled into the blood. Fortunately they do not exist forever, otherwise we would very soon become one solid block of antibody.

The job of lymphocytes is to police every corner of our body in search of undesirable invaders. The lymphocytes gain access to the body tissues by flowing round the body in the blood, from where they pass out to meander in close contact with the tissues' cells, which are bathed in a thin layer of fluid. They then find their way back into the blood via a second circulatory network, the lymphatic vessels (Figure 1). The lymphatic vessels empty their contents back into the blood circulation by joining with large veins behind the collarbone.

Scattered along the vessels of the lymphatic system are small swellings known as lymph nodes. Here, some lymphocytes rest, waiting to swing into action when infection strikes. You can locate some of the lymph nodes in your neck when you have a throat infection; the nodes feel hard (because they are now packed with active lymphocytes) and painful. Other places in the body where lymphocytes are found in high concentration are the bone marrow, where they originate, and the spleen and thymus, where some of them are "processed" (Figure 1).

TWO TYPES OF LYMPHOCYTES

One of the major milestones in modern immunology was the discovery seven years ago that the apparently homogenous population of lymphocytes is in fact made up of two distinct types—now known as T lymphocytes (or simply T cells) and B lymphocytes (B cells). Although T and B cells are both committed to defense against foreign invasion, they wield distinctly different weapons: the B cells are responsible for producing specific antibodies which disable invaders, while T cells inflict damage much more directly.

The dual systems of immunity—the humoral response (carried out by the B cells) and the cellular response (T cells)—perform slightly different jobs. Two years ago the different jobs could be stated very clearly: B cells unleash antibodies to destroy certain types of microorganisms, whereas T cells kill different types of microorganisms and also attack cancer and certain forms of parasites; T cells are also instrumental in rejecting organ transplants.

This simple duality is still basically valid, but the picture is now much more intricate than it was: T and B cells' functions are now known to overlap considerably; macrophages, another type of white blood cell, have shown themselves to be specifically involved in lymphocyte function; and at last scientists have recognized the intriguing phenomenon of cooperation between the two types of lymphocytes. We will go into these refinements later. First we should look more closely at the discovery of the basic duality in the immune system.

Nature Helps the Immunologists

As well as being noted for its amazing current rate of progress, powered by the tools of modern molecular biology, immunological research is peculiar in the close association between basic research and the problems of clinical medicine. In large measure this intimacy is due to the conviction of Dr. Robert Good that in order to learn the secrets of biology you have to listen to what Nature has to say. And Nature often makes its utterances through diseases that result from defects in the delicately balanced metabolic systems that make life possible. Good, who is currently director of the Memorial Sloan-Kettering Cancer Center in New York City, calls these diseases "experiments of Nature." It was by following a trail of experiments of Nature that Good and his colleagues discovered the dual nature of the immune response.

The story of the discovery illustrates so beautifully the potential of the immune system, and also its deficiencies, that it bears telling in some detail. In fact, it was mainly from the system's deficiencies—the so-called immunodeficiency diseases—that Good and his colleagues got their clues. Not that the story is a straightforward, uncomplicated elucidation of fact after fact. Far from it. Immunologists often found themselves up blind alleys, at times were totally baffled and at others were rescued by the most incredible pieces of good luck. It unfolded like any good scientific discovery. (Most of the time scientists prefer to imply that their discoveries are achieved by an ordered sequence of brilliant insights and careful deductions!)

The existence of the dual system of immunity emerged slowly over a long period, particularly over the past fifteen years or so. Throughout this time Good dissected vital clues from the experiments of Nature he so liked to discover and understand. Often he felt intuitively that the things the clinical situation seemed to imply were right, in spite of contradictory evidence in the research laboratory.

IMMUNOLOGY IN ITS INFANCY

After a difficult childhood—which involved a long and determined battle against paralysis in the legs, the residue of a serious illness—Good joined Berry Campbell at the University of Minnesota. Good was working "in a very desultory way" on herpes virus infections in the central nervous system. Although he quite enjoyed the pathology involved, he was bored by neurophysiology and was looking for something else to do. One night Fred Kolouch, another scientist at Minnesota, came to Good's laboratory and said, "Why don't you do something important? Come and help me work out my problem." Kolouch had been taking care of a patient with subacute bacterial endocarditis—a fatal infection involving Streptococcus viridans.

What intrigued Kolouch was that the patient's tissues were teeming with plasma cells (these cells were later discovered to be the descendants of B lymphocytes that manufacture antibodies). Four years earlier Kolouch had tried some experiments on rabbits to try to unravel the role of the plasma cells. Many people dismissed these cells as having no important function, as being merely passive. Kolouch was not so sure. He made a vaccine and injected it into rabbits. After an initial failure he induced an increase in the plasma cell population in the animals' bone marrow. This increase was accompanied by anaphylactic shock (a sort of allergic reaction), and Kolouch was not sure whether the increase in plasma cells was simply a secondary response. Nevertheless, Kolouch published a short note—in 1938—suggesting that plasma cells may be implicated in antibody formation during infections.

It was by helping Kolouch sort out some proper controls later that Good first got involved in immunology. This was Good's first encounter with an experiment of Nature—seeing a high level of plasma cells in a fatal infection. He analyzed Nature's experiment in the laboratory by inducing passive anaphylaxis in rabbits and discovered that the plasma cell level remained normal. Here was good evidence that plasma cells are involved in the immune response to infection.

A PLASMA CELL HUNTER

By 1949 Good had graduated from medical school and had completed house-officer training as a pediatrician. Meanwhile his dual life as a researcher and doctor continued and he had become an established "plasma cell hunter." Good was studying rheumatic fever in children, and he noticed that as the disease progressed the level of gamma globulin (protein antibodies) in the blood increased. In parallel with this he saw a build-up in the population of plasma cells—here was more evidence linking antibody production to plasma cells. In 1949 Good was invited to the Rockefeller

University, New York, to do a one-year research fellowship with Maclyn McCarty. It was while he was at the Rockefeller for that year that Good developed a deep love for New York, an affection that played a large part in persuading him eventually to break his long association with the University of Minnesota.

During his year at the Rockefeller, Good met Henry Kunkel. Kunkel wanted to get access to some myeloma patients (who have a tumor of the plasma cell system) so he could study the protein products of the plasma cells. As an indoctrinated plasma cell hunter, Good was just the man to help out Kunkel with his problem. So by one of those quirks of fate the right two men came together in the same place at the same time. From their brief association sprang all the work that was to lead to the detailed molecular description of protein antibodies that earned Gerald Edelman (of the Rockefeller University) and Rodney Porter (of Oxford) joint shares in the 1972 Nobel Prize for Medicine.

The discovery of antibody structure began with Good drawing samples of blood from myeloma patients and Kunkel isolating the gamma globulins and doing beautiful immuno-chemical analysis of these proteins. Both men were to learn a lot from the experiment, but in very different ways. Kunkel found that plasma cells manufactured a series of proteins that were quite distinct from each other, yet closely related. This turned out to be the large family of protein antibodies with which we are so familiar today. While Kunkel was "opening the Pandora's box," Good was learning a great deal simply by talking to his patients, something he had to do because he was sticking needles into their arms to get blood, but also something he always makes a point of doing anyway.

While he was talking to his myeloma patients Good learned that they had severe problems with infection. This puzzled him because he knew the patients had lots of plasma cells (and therefore antibody) in their blood. Plasma cells are designed to fight infection, so why did these patients have more than their fair share of infections? (Remember, the twin arms of the immune system were nowhere in sight in 1949.)

THE FIRST GLIMMERINGS OF DUALITY

Meanwhile, Good was doing what he considered was a rather pedestrian job that he thought would please his boss McCarty. Some time earlier McCarty had crystallized a so-called C-reactive protein, a protein that appears at the beginning of acute infection and disappears later on. Good went in search of a suitable source, which turned out to be Hodgkin's disease patients (this is a tumor of certain lymph nodes, which are part of the immune system). Once again Good came into close contact with patients while he was collecting samples for McCarty to analyze. And once again he discovered that these patients also had problems with infections, but their infections were different from the myeloma patients'. People with Hodgkin's disease were particularly susceptible to low-grade infections, whereas myeloma was associated with a vulnerability to high-grade pathogens. What could it mean? Good also suspected that delayed-type hypersensitivity (which we now know to involve cellular immunity) was not linked to antibody production. In retrospect these were the first glimmerings of the now well-established dual immune systems. But at the time—1950—"it was all very confusing." "It was simply a clinical observation," Good now says, "but it was certainly a thorn in my side."

When he went back to Minnesota—in 1950—Good was joined by Lewis Thomas, who is now the new president of the Memorial Sloan-Kettering Cancer Center. By 1952 they were doing what turned out to be important work on agammaglobulinemia (no antibodies in the blood), though they did not recognize it at the time. Good had some patients who were extraordinarily susceptible to infections, so he was looking at their white blood cells to try to find out why. The clue came when Ogden Bruton published a paper in the *Pediatric Journal* describing a boy in Virginia who was unable to defend himself against high-grade pathogens. This boy had no plasma cells and very little gamma globulin in his blood. Good immediately looked at his own patients and found they were just like Bruton's—they also lacked plasma cells.

More pointers to the dual immune system came when Good discovered that these agammaglobulinemic patients were quite capable of developing delayed-type hypersensitivity reactions and could also reject foreign skin grafts (both of these are mediated mainly by the cellular immune system). "But it was all still a great haze and I didn't begin to express the ideas about two systems clearly until three years later [1955]."

IMMUNOLOGICAL DUO: THYMUS AND BURSA

Yet another experiment of Nature presented itself in 1952. One of the patients Good studied with Richard Varco had broad-based immunodeficiency together with a large tumor of the thymus gland (which is just behind the breastbone). This prompted him to wonder—as other people had—what role the thymus gland might play in immunity. Having been presented with a model by Nature, Good tried to simulate it in the research laboratory. He took out the thymus from four-week-old rabbits to see if it affected the animals' immune competence. It did not do a thing. Good was puzzled. But he was so convinced that there must be something important in the clinical observation that he wrote a paper saying that the experiment of Nature must be significant and that the laboratory equipment must be at fault.

Good had to wait until 1959 before he got any real clue about what it all meant. But because of the perhaps understandable lack of judgment of the prestigious American journal *Science,* the clue had languished unheeded in an obscure back alley of the scientific press. In the mid-1950s Bruce Glick, a graduate student at Ohio State University, was trying to discover the function of a tiny gland—the bursa

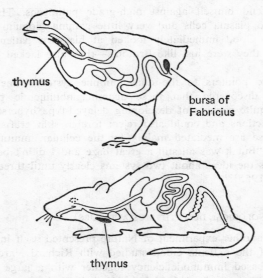

Figure 2. Birds have both a thymus and a bursa of Fabricius, but mammals have only a thymus.

of Fabricius (see Figure 2)—at the end of a chick's alimentary canal. Glick's teacher had told him that if he could discover what the gland did he would be a famous man. Glick removed the bursa from chicks of all ages and observed them to see what effect it had. As far as he could see nothing happened. He was getting nowhere. Meanwhile he was supposed to be teaching a short course on the immune response, but because he had already done it once he sloughed the job to Timothy Chang, another graduate student.

While he was preparing the class demonstration, Chang made the mistake of using a chick that had been bursectomized immediately after hatching; he thought it was a normal bird. To his great embarrassment he was unable to induce an immune response in the class demonstration. But Glick was delighted because he now had a function for his pet gland—it must be involved in immunity. They tried to get the observation published in *Science,* but the journal dismissed it as "being of no general interest." Much discouraged, Glick published it in *Poultry Science,* where it lay unnoticed for several years until Harold Wolff, a friend of Good's, came across it in 1959.

Wolff had developed elegant techniques for measuring protein in chicken blood. So he applied his methods to a chick bursectomized at hatching and discovered that the antibody level was disastrously low. He told Good, who became very excited about it all. "It was a bolt out of the blue," Good says. The excitement in the Minnesota lab was tremendous. If the bursa has to be removed at hatching to have any effect on immunity the thymus might have to be removed immediately after birth. Was this what was wrong with the previous thymectomy experiments all those years before? To check they thymectomized "hot little newborn rabbits." It worked. The animals' immune response was blunted and in a very selected way. Thymectomized rabbits could manufacture some antibodies pretty well, but they were unable to reject foreign grafts or develop delayed-type hypersensitivity reactions. Here at last was a good demonstration of the dual systems of immunity.

By one of those uncanny coincidences that so often occur in research, at least three and possibly four groups lit upon the importance of the thymus at the same time. Jaques Miller at the Chester Beatty Research Institute in London came up with the same conclusion as Good, but from an entirely different direction. Macfarlane Burnet's group in Australia and Bernard Waksman's group at Harvard were also on to it.

Although the haze was beginning to lift from the dual nature of the immune system, it was not cleared. Good decided to concentrate on chicks for a bit because the two central lymphoid systems were readily accessible there. By 1965 he had learned a lot. The bursa is needed for the development of germinal centers in lymph nodes that give rise to plasma cells and one population of lymphocytes, both of which can produce antibodies. The thymus, however, is responsible for generating a population of lymphocytes which mediate the cellular response. Max Cooper, a colleague of Good's, presented all this at a clinical meeting in 1965. He said the agammaglobulinemia patients are just like bursectomized animals. Immediately a man ran from his seat to the microphone and shouted, "That's it; that's exactly what we've been seeing in Philadelphia." The man, Angello Di George, was working with children who lacked thymuses. He knew they had plenty of antibodies, but they still could not live. The reason was now obvious to him—they lacked the cellular arm of the immune defense.

REPAIRING IMMUNODEFICIENCY

Gradually immunologists were beginning to dissect the defense system and could contemplate selective repairs in patients with certain types of immunodeficiencies. At a conference in 1967 on immunodeficiencies, the participants decided that there ought to be two procedures for correcting deficiencies: thymus transplant for Di George type patients, and bone marrow transplant for combined immunodeficiency. Bill Cleveland of Miami succeeded in curing the cellular immunodeficiency by transplanting fetal thymus membranes into a patient with Di George's syndrome. Good and his colleagues tried the bone marrow transplant, but ran into difficulties.

The first bone marrow transplant Good tried was on a little boy dying of combined immunodeficiency; he could not defend himself against any infection. The Minnesota team used fetal liver as a substitute for bone marrow, and did a thymus transplant as well. The immune system was repaired perfectly but the boy died because the graft had attacked the host tissues—a graft-versus-host reaction. Good was extremely discouraged by this failure. But sitting half dozing one night—"I become a pumpkin about eleven-thirty" —the answer suddenly came to him. It was 1:20 A.M. when Good rushed to the telephone to tell his colleagues Dick Hong and Ed Yunis. They were sure he was right. Good was so confident that with Hong he wrote a paper telling everyone how to do it. The trick, he guessed, was to match donor and recipient with respect to their major histocompatibility components.

A few months later (in 1968) a suitable case arrived, the procedure was carried out and the patient was cured. The patient was the little boy whose dramatic rescue opened this book.

Good is now trying to dissect out the molecular components of the immune system. He's not daunted by this challenge because he places great faith in the powerful analytical techniques that are now available. "It took Wilfred Stein and Stanford Moore longer than ten years in the 1950s to get an amino acid sequence of a protein; it now takes seventy minutes. With the sort of methodology we have today the word 'factor' is obsolete. You can now characterize and quantify substances very rapidly. This is part of a great scientific revolution."

THE LYMPHOCYTES ARE CHRISTENED

By 1969, then, the two divisions of the immune system were revealed. It was also in that year that the terms T and B lymphocytes were coined. Ivan Roitt, professor of immunology at the Middlesex Hospital Medical School, London, England, was lying in bed one January morning wrestling with a bout of English flu. To pass the time he was mentally juggling with these new discoveries when the terms came to him—T for thymus and B for bursa. The names stuck and they work very well, except for one awkward fact: mammals do not have a bursa!

The search for the mammalian equivalent of the bursa has become frustrating and unrewarding. Some people suggest that Peyer's patches (lymphoid tissue in the lower part of the intestine) might do for mammals what the bursa does for the birds. Others think the appendix might be implicated. But no one has any really good evidence. It may be that in mammals B lymphocytes do not need to be processed by a bursa-like organ. For instance, Martin Raff of University

College, London, thinks that the bone marrow itself may do the job of the bursa. It is ironic that the discovery of the dual system in mammals (which is undisputed) depended on the experimental removal of an organ that is found only in birds!

The Lymphocytes' Journey

We can now sketch the life history of T and B lymphocytes. Both types start life as stem cells in the bone marrow. From there some go to the thymus, where they are exposed to a chemical—thymic hormone—that speeds the maturation of the T cell function. There is a great deal of cell proliferation and destruction in the thymus, and only a small proportion of the cells in that organ ever escape from it. Those that do get out circulate through the blood and the lymph; some of them spend periods in the lymph nodes. The circulating T lymphocytes, often called the small lymphocytes, live many years, and are constantly on the lookout for foreign invaders.

Lymphocytes destined to be B cells are processed by the bursa or its mammalian equivalent and then preferentially reside in the lymph nodes, though a small proportion do circulate in the blood. The proportion of T to B cells in the blood is eight to two; the B cells dominate in the lymph nodes (Figure 3).

For the lymphocyte to be able to mediate recognition, memory and specificity, it must have some considerable degree of sophistication which so far we have not considered. Since "the new immunology" is the child of molecular biology, it is not surprising to find that the lymphocytes' function rests on the molecular sophistication invested in the protein molecules so closely associated with lymphocytes: the antibodies. Before discussing the mechanics of the immune responses as a whole (Chapter 5), we need to examine the molecular mechanisms that lie behind the recognition functions of antibodies.

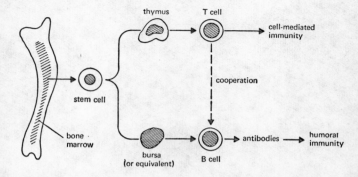

Figure 3. THE TWIN ARMS OF IMMUNITY: Some stem cells from the bone marrow pass through the thymus, where they mature into T cells which mediate cellular immunity; others are processed by the bursa (or its equivalent) and become B cells which are capable of producing large quantities of antibodies.

2. Locks and Keys of Immunity

"Antibodies occupy a central place in the science of immunology for an obvious reason: they are the protein molecules responsible for the recognition of foreign molecules or antigens."

Gerald Edelman (of the Rockefeller University, New York) made this statement at the end of 1972 as part of a lecture he gave when he received science's greatest accolade—the Nobel Prize. In that year Edelman shared the Nobel Prize for Medicine with Rodney Porter (of Oxford University) for their separate efforts in elucidating the molecular structure of antibodies. Their success, in what Edelman describes as the first project of molecular immunology, laid the foundations for a rational interpretation of the molecular sophistication of the immune response carried out by lymphocytes.

The Discovery of Antibodies

Antibodies were first realized to be part of the body's natural defense mechanisms before the end of the last century, though at the time scientists did not know what they were. In 1890, Emil von Behring and Shibasaburo Kitazato discovered that substances called *Antikörper* appeared in the blood of animals when they suffered an infection. One year later, on Christmas Eve, von Behring put his new knowledge to clinical test in a dramatic experiment.

A little German girl lay in a Berlin clinic teetering on the brink of death. She was dying from diphtheria. There was nothing anyone could do. Von Behring knew that his *Antikörper* were capable of neutralizing poisons, so he decided to risk a last-resort attempt to save the girl's life. The German scientist ordered that a sheep be infected with the diphtheria bacterium and that the animal's blood, which contained the natural protective substances, should be collected. When he had enough sheep serum (that is, blood with the red cells removed) containing the *Antikörper* he arranged for it to be injected into the little girl. It worked. Within hours the dying child began to recover.

This courageous gamble, which marked the first application of scientific medicine to the cure of an acute infectious disease, earned von Behring the 1901 Nobel Prize for Medicine. The German scientist had pioneered what we now call passive immunity: the girl was able to fight the infection using immune weapons (the sheep's antibodies) she herself had not manufactured. Passive immunity is resorted to when an acute situation develops in which there is no time to stimulate a normal immune response.

Antigens

What is it then that stimulates the immune system—the lymphocytes—to produce antibodies? The diphtheria bacteria that Behring injected into his sheep can do it. So too can the vaccinia viruses that Edward Jenner used to induce immunity against smallpox. Because these organisms *generate* antibody manufacture, they are called antigens. But an antigen does not have to be either a virus or a bacterium. Many very different molecules are potentially antigenic, that is, capable of being recognized by lymphocytes' surveillance systems.

The important thing to remember about molecules—whether they are proteins, fats or carbohydrates—is that in general they have specific shapes. A protein molecule, which is a string of several hundred amino acids linked together, wraps itself up in a very specific conformation which is determined by the sequence of amino acids in the chain.

This means that in a protein that forms itself roughly into a sphere, as many of them do, some amino acids are exposed on the outside as bumps and ridges, while others are hidden in the center of the sphere.

Proteins are very potent antigens, but the antibodies that react with them do not recognize the protein molecule as a whole. There are certain small areas on the molecule—made up of three to ten amino acids—known as antigenic determinants. It is an antigenic determinant that an antibody recognizes. Any large protein molecule therefore has a number of antigenic determinants on its exposed surfaces, each of which may be recognized by an antibody. Similarly, a large carbohydrate molecule can sport an array of antigenic determinants. An antigenic determinant is a molecule or portion of a molecule capable of binding firmly to the combining site of an antibody; an antigen is a molecule containing one or more antigenic determinants.

Not wishing to leave everything to Nature, scientists have manufactured their own antigens. They have found that the immune system is capable of reacting to almost any kind of non-natural molecule, even very small ones. These small synthetic antigens are known as haptens. But because they are so small they are unable to provoke an immune reaction unless they are bound to a larger carrier molecule.

Immunogenicity

This brings us to an important distinction in the relationship between foreign molecules and the immune system. The vaccinia virus, which carries a number of proteins on its surface, provokes an immune response (antibody production) when it is injected into an animal—it is said to be immunogenic. A small hapten molecule, which is antigenic in that it can be recognized by the appropriate antibody molecule if it is present, provokes no immune response—it is not immunogenic. The distinction between antigenic and immunogenic is therefore an important one. Immunogenicity involves two stages: recognition of an antigen by an antibody, followed by the triggering of an immune response. An antigen is not necessarily an immunogen. We will see later why this is so when we talk about cooperation in the immune response.

LOCKS AND KEYS

So far we have said that antibodies recognize antigens (or rather the determinants on them), but in our definition we used the term "binding" in referring to the reaction between antigens and antibodies. Humans recognize each other by *looking* for characteristic shapes and forms (usually in the face). Antibodies also use shape and form to recognize molecules, but obviously they cannot *see* them. Instead they use a lock-and-key system in which an antigen of a particular shape slots perfectly into a combining site on the antibody molecule (Figure 4).

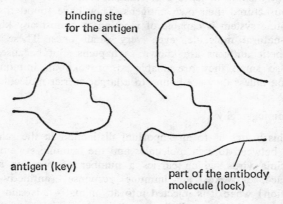

binding site
for the antigen

antigen (key)

part of the antibody
molecule (lock)

Figure 4. The specific shape of an antigen fits into a complementary shape on an antibody molecule.

Man's immune machinery is capable of reacting to (that is, recognizing and responding to) at least 100,000 different antigens. This implies that we must have the ability to synthesize an equal number of antibodies, each of which has a combining site whose shape matches one of the antigenic determinants. The mechanism behind this generation of diversity—or GOD as immunologists quip—has been one of the major puzzles of antibody research for a very long time. And it is one of the problems that has been greatly illuminated by Edelman's and Porter's achievements in working out the structure of antibodies, as we shall see in the following chapter.

What then is the connection between an antibody recognizing an invading antigen and the production of more antibody as a response? First, it is the B cells (or rather their progeny, the plasma cells) that manufacture antibodies on a big scale. Sitting on the surface of the lymphocyte are antibody molecules—100,000 of them—acting as lookouts for the appropriate antigen (Figure 5). All the antibody

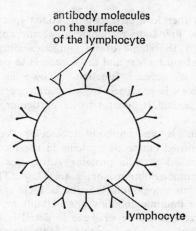

antibody molecules
on the surface
of the lymphocyte

lymphocyte

Figure 5. Y-shaped antibody molecules are arranged on the lymphocyte surface as receptors for antigens.

molecules on any one B cell surface are the same, and the antibodies produced by the cell when it is stimulated are all identical to the ones acting as surface receptors. In other words, any particular B cell (and its progeny) deals in only one type of antibody which reacts with just one type of antigenic determinant. In a later chapter we will examine the dynamics of antibody production, and the key supporting role performed by T cells.

Five Classes of Antibody

The millions of different antibodies which correspond to an equal number of antigenic determinants can be categorized into five major classes: G, M, A, D and E. These class divisions are not made on the type of antigen responded to; rather they are determined by the molecular structure of the antibodies themselves. These structural differences influence the type of defensive reaction the particular antibody exerts.

Antibodies therefore have two functions specified by their structure: the first is to recognize a specific antigen (this is determined by the shape of its antigen-binding site and is unique to that antibody); and the second is to perform a particular type of defense function (known as the effector function) which is governed by a separate part of the antibody molecule and is general to its particular class (G, M etc.).

What then is an antibody molecule? Von Behring's *Antikörper* turned out to be proteins in the blood associated with the so-called globulin proteins. Antibodies are therefore known as immunoglobulins, or Ig for short. The shorthand for the five immunoglobulin classes is IgG, IgM, IgA, IgD and IgE. The immunoglobulins are all built on basically the same structure (which we shall see in detail in the following chapter). They are large proteins containing about 1,330 amino acids in their chains.

CLASS DIFFERENCES

The most primitive of all the antibodies is IgM, and it is the first to be produced in response to a challenge by antigen that gets into the blood. Compared with IgG, the avidity with which IgM binds with its antigens is fairly low, reflecting perhaps its more lowly position in the evolutionary scale. IgM is curious in that, unlike the other antibodies, it goes around in fives—five molecules are linked together to form what is called a pentamer. In spite of, or perhaps because of, this odd arrangement, IgM is particularly efficient at dealing with invading bacteria. The antibody binds with antigenic determinants on the bacterium's surface and then, with the help of another set of proteins that circulate in the blood (known as the complement system), it punches holes in the organism's membrane, thus destroying it. The surface of a bacterium that has been attacked by antibody aided by complement looks like a crater-covered battlefield.

The presence of IgM on bacterial membranes also stirs into action another set of cells called macrophages. These cells can devour invading bacteria and destroy them, but without a layer of antibody on the target organism they are not very efficient. The buttering of bacteria with antibody so as to whet the appetite of macrophages is known as opsonization. Like all antibodies, IgM can also damage bacteria simply by binding to and blocking important areas on the organism's outer membrane. IgM production following infection in the blood and surrounding tissues can be thought of as the panic button response: it is quick, but lacks tight specificity.

As an infection continues, antibody production switches to IgG, the major mammalian antibody. Although IgG is less efficient than IgM at fixing complement (as the reaction is called), the IgGs produced are much more specific to the invading antigens. Once manufactured and released into the blood, IgG survives for many weeks; IgM lasts for only one sixth as long as its more sophisticated successor. Because of its comparative longevity, IgG confers "medium-term" immunity in an individual. (We shall see later that "long-term" immunity, lasting a lifetime perhaps, is the responsibility of a form of lymphocyte known as memory cells.)

One important consequence of the bulk structure of IgG

(that is, the portion not responsible for binding antigens) is that it is able to cross certain cell barriers. IgG is the only antibody class that can pass across the placenta and reach the developing fetus. This export of antibody from mother to unborn child is crucial because until the fetus is twenty weeks old it is unable to produce any type of antibody. At this stage, and for several weeks after its birth, the child is dependent on passive immunity (from its mother) for protection against any kind of antigen. Maternal milk also contains IgG, and this is one reason for encouraging a mother to breast-feed for up to two months after the birth. After that the baby begins to marshal its own immune defenses. Finally, IgG also has the distinction of being the most studied class of antibody. It was on IgG that Porter and Edelman did all their major structural analysis.

Not only does IgG have the distinction of being the major mammalian antibody, it also has the unusual feature of coming in four different forms, denoted IgG1, IgG2, IgG3 and IgG4. IgG2–4 are minor structural variations of IgG1, which is by far the most predominant form. They all carry out roughly the same functions, except that IgG2 and 4 cannot fix complement, and that IgG3 has a much shorter life span than its cousins.

Both IgM and IgG defend us against organisms (bacteria and viruses) and toxins (which are poisons produced by some bacteria) that manage to get into the body and come in close and threatening contact with our tissues. Both types of antibody exploit complement fixation, opsonization and critical area blocking in their reactions to antigen challenge. A third class of antibody, IgA, acts as a barrier against pathogenic organisms actually entering our body. The lining of the intestine contains large numbers of IgA-producing cells. The antibody they manufacture is released into the gut where it forms an "antiseptic paint," as Macfarlane Burnet calls it, in the sticky mucus that lines the wall of the intestine.

The content of our gut is potentially harmful to us. It contains many bacteria that are important in digesting food and providing important vitamins. But if they escape from the gut and find their way into the blood they can cause serious blood poisoning, or septicemia. The IgA barrier helps prevent this. This secretory antibody, as it is sometimes called, patrols all the wet, vulnerable surfaces of our body: for instance, it is found in the lining of the respiratory tract, in the gut, in saliva, in tears and in sweat. Once again, it is the bulk structure of the IgA class that confers on it this particular function.

IgE is better known for its nuisance than for its beneficial attributes. This antibody is responsible for triggering the unpleasant effects of allergy and asthma. IgE molecules bind (by their non-antigen-binding areas) to the surface of mast cells. These cells contain histamine, which, as every hay fever sufferer who pops dozens of antihistamine pills down his throat every summer knows, causes unpleasant irritation to the eyes and nose. When an allergen—that is, a molecule or particle (such as pollen) that triggers an allergy—binds to the antigen-binding site of an IgE molecule sitting on a mast cell, the histamine is released into the blood. Nature would have been totally mad, or just perverse, to have invented an antibody which has only nuisance value. Some researchers have observed that the level of IgE in the blood rises when an animal is invaded by parasites. One might infer therefore that IgE is designed to combat parasites, but this remains to be proved.

If IgE is a bit of a puzzle, IgD is a total mystery. No one has any really good idea of what it does. Whatever it does, it cannot be a major activity because the amount in the blood is very low (Table 1).

Table 1   Class differences in antibodies

Immunoglobulin class	Amount in serum	% in the serum	Approximate half-life
IgG	12.0 mgs/ml	45	23.0 days
IgA	3.5 mgs/ml	42	5.8
IgM	1.2 mgs/ml	76	5.1
IgD	0.03 mgs/ml	75	2.8
IgE	0.0000105 mgs/ml	51	2.3

Maturation of Antibody Production

The capacity to manufacture immunoglobulins begins at twenty weeks of gestation. At this time a developing fetus can produce IgM and IgA if severely challenged by antigen. The fetus cannot make its own IgG, possibly because its production is inhibited by the presence of its mother's (inhibition by negative feedback). Although a baby is born with a normal adult level of IgG in its blood (from its mother), this rapidly falls off and does not resume adult measures again until about four years of age. Blood levels of IgM take between one to two years to become "adult," while for secretory IgA maturation takes just a few months.

The immunoglobulins have preferences about the part of the body they inhabit. IgM and IgD are preferentially localized within the circulatory systems, whereas the others are more evenly distributed throughout the body. This does not hold for secretory IgA, which finds itself almost totally "outside" the body on wet surfaces.

Primary and Secondary Responses

When an animal is challenged with antigen it has never encountered before, one sees a curious switch in antibody production. First the animal's immune system takes a while to get tooled up to respond, and when it does it produces IgM antibodies. The presence of a specific IgM in the blood stimulates more production of the same antibody—this is one of the rare examples in biology of positive feedback. Positive feedback can bring about an unstable situation, with the whole system accelerating faster and faster.

Disaster is averted with this system because very soon the cells that were synthesizing IgM switch to producing IgG. (Remember, the two classes of antibody can react with exactly the same antigens.) While there is still enough antigen in the body to mop up the IgG released, the blood level of that specific IgG remains low. But once the antigen has been removed IgG begins to build up. It is this build-up that now switches off the antibody production—a very effective control system known as negative feedback (Figure 6). The T cells may also play an as yet unraveled role in switching off antibody production.

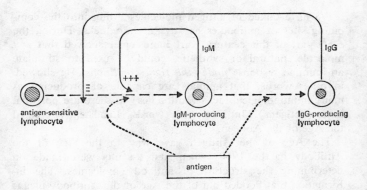

Figure 6. NEGATIVE FEEDBACK CONTROL OF ANTIBODY PRODUCTION: Antigen promotes the conversion of antigen-sensitive cells into IgM-producing cells, and the maturation of the latter into IgG-producing cells. IgM antibody enhances the formation of IgM-producing cells (+++), whereas IgG inhibits it (≡). IgG inhibition can operate only when there is excess antibody available (that is, when the antigen is beginning to be mopped up).

This response to a new antigen—a lag period for tooling up, IgM production, followed by IgG—is known as the primary response. When an animal is challenged a second time the reaction is much more swift. In the secondary response antibody production starts immediately, and the IgM stage is bypassed altogether; only IgG is produced as the major reaction. (In fact, in any antigen challenge all antibodies are produced to some extent, with the exception of IgM in a secondary response.) The basis of the rapid secondary response is immunological memory which is mediated by descendants of B cells known as memory cells. The

system remembers all the antigens it has met and is ready
for them the next time. We will discuss the cellular mechanisms of immunological memory in a later chapter.

The Age of the Antibody

We have talked of antigen molecules fitting into the combining sites of antibodies as keys fit into locks. During the
early part of this century Karl Landsteiner showed that any
molecule, natural or synthetic, could be used to stimulate
an immune response *under the right conditions*. He showed,
in other words, that animals are capable of producing as
many immunological locks (antibodies) as there are potential
keys (antigens). In Edelman's words, Landsteiner created
the Age of the Antigen.

The Age of the Antigen gave way to the Age of the
Antibody in the 1960s when first assaults were made on
determining the structure of antibody molecules. The information that flooded out of the Age of the Antibody means
that many of the most fundamental problems of immunology
can be answered. Prominent among these problems is the
mechanisms behind the B lymphocytes' ability to produce
such a vast range of immunological locks, the vast majority of which will never be called upon to go into action.

THE ORIGIN OF DIVERSITY

This phenomenon of antibody diversity stems ultimately
from how an individual specific antibody molecule is manufactured. Antibodies are protein molecules, so one can draw
on the fruits of molecular biology to describe their production. Very briefly, the information for making a protein is
stored in the nucleic acid structure of the genes (DNA).
This information is first transcribed into a message (messenger
RNA) that the cell's manufacturing machinery can understand, and then the protein is assembled by stringing together
amino acids in the order specified by the message (Figure 7).

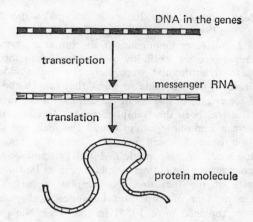

Figure 7. A scheme for the transcription of the codes stored in DNA into RNA messages which are then translated into protein molecules.

With the benefit of this and other knowledge from the molecular biologists we know that the final specific shape of a protein molecule is determined solely by the sequence of amino acids from which it is made. But when scientists first started thinking about antibody manufacture molecular biology was a thing of the future.

EARLY THEORIES

Paul Ehrlich, the great German scientist, proposed the first important theory of antibody formation in 1897. His "side-chain" theory stated that antigens encountered chemical groupings, or side-chains, in cells and that occasionally there was a perfect fit between the antigen and the side-chain. Once disturbed in this way the cell would manufacture more of that specific side-chain to make up for the ones lost. Ehrlich called these side-chains antitoxins. Although this idea is clearly not tenable it does contain the seeds of a major tenet

of modern immunology: that cells can make specific antibodies before they encounter the specific antigen.

When Landsteiner demonstrated the immune system's immense repertoire of antibody production, the notion that
antibodies (or antitoxins) were mere chemical accidents lost
favor. Instead, people came to think that maybe the antigen
induced some kind of change in the cell's synthetic machinery.
Out of this was born the "template theory." Felix Haurowitz,
an American immunologist, proposed the idea and said that
an antigen entered a cell where it formed a template on
which the antibody molecule folded itself; an antibody directly
complementary to the antigen would therefore be formed.

In spite of the fact that the template theory failed to
explain a number of important immunological phenomena,
it was not replaced until 1955. In that year Niels Jerne, a
Danish immunologist, presented his "natural selection
theory," which said that the blood contains a vast range of
natural antibody molecules. An antigen entering the blood is
bound to meet an antibody to which it fits. When this happens the united pair are taken up by a phagocytic cell where-
upon the antibody acts as a template for its own reproduction.

CLONAL SELECTION

Two years later, in 1957, Jerne's theory was superseded
by the "clonal selection theory," an idea that has come to
be verified and accepted. The notion was born twice, independently. Sir Frank Macfarlane Burnet, the great Australian immunologist, and David Talmage, of the University
of Colorado, both had the same idea at the same time, one
of those curious coincidences in the development of science.
Like Jerne they envisaged a low level of antibodies circulating in the blood, but they placed emphasis on the antibody-
producing cells themselves rather than their products.

The clonal selection theory proposes that an unstimulated
animal has in it a vast range of antibody-producing cells
(B lymphocytes) that are already committed to respond to
a particular antigen. Once a lymphocyte encounters its

specific antigen it proliferates, producing a large number
of progeny all committed to producing the specific antibody
(Figure 8). (Antibody production is in fact more com-

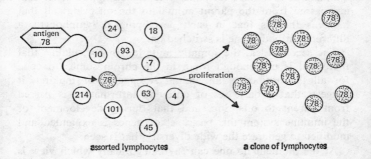

Figure 8. CLONAL SELECTION: The body contains small numbers
of different lymphocytes capable of manufacturing different antibodies (denoted by the numbers). When a specific antigen encounters its corresponding lymphocyte, that lymphocyte is stimulated to proliferate, thus producing a clone of identical cells.

plicated than that, as we shall see in the next chapter. But
the theory still holds.) A clone is a group of cells all originat-
ing from the same parent cell, hence the term "clonal selection." The group of cells is "selected" out by the specificity
of the antigen. Appropriately enough it was Gus Nossal,
the man who succeeded Burnet as director of the Walter
and Eliza Hall Institute of Medical Research in Australia,
who provided much of the evidence to show that indeed all
the progeny of a proliferating cell do indeed manufacture
the same specific antibody as the parent cell.

TWO THEORIES OF DIVERSITY

Having seen that an animal has the potential to manufacture
antibodies to any antigen presented to it (by selecting the
appropriate pre-existing clone), we are forced to come back
to the question of what gives rise to the generation of

diversity—the GOD—of antibody formation. There are two main explanations offered. The first, the germ line theory, says that the information to code for all the antibodies an animal will ever need to make is contained in the genes that are passed from the parent animal to the offspring; all that happens then is that in each developing B lymphocyte, a different antibody gene is switched on.

The second idea, the somatic mutation theory, claims that there just is not enough room in the chromosomes to code for all the antibodies an animal is capable of making; it suggests that a basic set of antibody information is passed from parent to offspring, and that during development of the immune system this basic set of genes is expanded and modified to generate the wide diversity that is seen.

At the moment no one can say categorically which view is correct. That day will probably not be possible until one can actually count the number of antibody genes passed from parent to offspring. Nevertheless, the new knowledge about antibody structure has given keen insights into the basis of the diversity, if not its origin. It also elucidated the nature of the two functions of antibodies (antigen-binding and effector function), as well as giving clues about the molecular evolution of the antibodies themselves. We should therefore now follow the remarkable story of this, the first major project of molecular immunology.

3. Birth of Molecular Immunology

The Age of the Antigen was born out of the marriage between immunology and chemistry, under the guidance of Karl Landsteiner. The Age of the Antibody was created from the union between immunology and molecular biology, carefully nurtured by Gerald Edelman and Rodney Porter.

When the separate brilliance of two research teams—Edelman's in New York and Porter's in Oxford—combined to solve the details of antibody structure, the science of immunology underwent a major revolution, after which it can never be the same again: some of the current notions were provided with rationale at the molecular level; novel insights had to be coped with and assimilated into people's thinking; and, most important of all, the once dim prospect of finely tuning the immunological response at last came close to realization. We should follow this story because it ranks among the most important in the pages of the history of immunology. But first we will cheat a little and take a look at a chemical structure that less than five years ago was not known to a single person in the whole world—an immunoglobulin.

Antibody Structure

Immunoglobulins are proteins. Many protein molecules are made up of a single long chain of amino acids strung together. But the immunoglobulins are slightly different from this simple arrangement. Every single immunoglobulin molecule is made up of four separate protein chains joined together with special bonds. The four chains are in fact two pairs: one pair is short and is called the light chains, while the other is much longer and is known as the heavy chains. Overall, the molecule is Y-shaped (Figure 9).

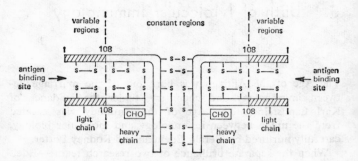

Figure 9. THE STRUCTURE OF AN ANTIBODY MOLECULE: The four-chain arrangement (two light and two heavy) can be easily seen. The shaded area represents the variable portion of the chains.

Each light chain has about 220 amino acids strung in a line, while each heavy chain has twice that number. The light and heavy chains have one structural characteristic in common: part of the chain is constant while the rest is variable. What does this mean?

CONSTANT STRUCTURES

First, let us examine the heavy chain. If we analyze the constant regions of a whole range of antibodies of, say, the IgG class we find that the sequence of amino acids in them is the same. But the arrangement of amino acids at the end of the heavy chains in these IgGs—that is, in the variable regions—is different for every particular specific antibody. Hence the names, variable and constant regions. Turning now to the other immunoglobulin classes, we find that the constant regions of the heavy chains of all IgM antibodies are identical, those for IgE are identical and so on. In other words, it is the constant region, or heavy chains, that determine the class of antibody. The heavy chains are therefore designated by the Greek letters corresponding to G, M, A, D and E: γ, μ, a, δ, ϵ.

The structure of the constant region of the heavy chains governs the effector regions of the different antibody classes. It explains why, for instance, IgG passes across the placenta to the developing baby, why IgM is so good at fixing complement, why IgA can be secreted onto wet membranes and why IgE binds itself to mast cells.

VARIABLE STRUCTURES

What then of the variable region on the heavy chain? It is the long list of variations in amino acid sequences found in this area between different antibodies that is responsible at least in part for providing the specific binding site for a particular antibody. Also contributing to the unique nature of antigen-specific binding sites is the variable region of the light chain. We shall see later how the combination of two variable regions (one from the heavy chain, the other from the light) greatly increases the possible number of combining sites. Between fifteen and twenty amino acids—from variable regions of both the light and heavy chains—contribute directly to creating the specific shape and form of the antigen-binding site. Probably many more amino acids contribute subtly to the binding site without being directly involved.

There are two classes of light chain, lambda and kappa. (As with the heavy chains, the constant region determines the class.) As shown in Figure 9 the first 108 amino acids make up the variable regions of both the light and heavy chains. When Edelman and his colleagues looked at the different permutations possible in the variable regions they found that some areas are more variable than others. There are three areas, known as hypervariable regions, in which the frequency and range of amino acid substitutions are greater than in the rest of the region. This variable variability also holds for the heavy chains. Finally, kappa light chains can be divided into three subgroups, according to the over-all basic pattern of the amino acid sequences in the variable region, and lambda into five. A given antibody has either kappa or lambda light chains, not a mixture of the two.

ANTIGEN-BINDING SITES

We see therefore that every antibody molecule has two antigen-binding sites, one at each end of the Y. These two sites in any particular antibody molecule are always identical, that is, they bind the same antigen. Every individual antibody carries two identical heavy chains (which determine the Ig class, and therefore the effector function) linked to two identical light chains (which specifies the antigen which the molecule recognizes). Lambda and kappa light chains can be associated with any class of heavy chain.

The Beginning of the Story

If that is the end product of the story, how did it begin? By the end of the 1950s antibodies were acknowledged to be of some importance in immunology, and people had quite a few guesses about what they could do. Landsteiner, for instance, had shown that antibodies operate by molecular complementarity; that is, the antigen "fits" into a specific site on the antibody. And there was good evidence that each antibody molecule had two binding sites. Immunologists knew too that as a group immunoglobulins were extraordinarily heterogeneous, that they came in many different forms.

Two men, Porter and Edelman, realized that without a detailed picture of antibody structure immunologists were going to be stuck. So, in their different ways, they set about tackling what by any standards was an enormous task. Porter did his apprenticeship with Fred Sanger, the Nobel Prize winner from Cambridge. While he was with Sanger, Porter learned two vital tricks: one, how to deal with proteins, and two, how to stick at a seemingly impossible task. (Sanger had been awarded his prize for his pioneering efforts on sequencing amino acids in proteins.)

When Porter moved to the National Institute for Medical Research in London he already had the idea of smashing up the antibody molecule to find out which bit did the antigen binding, that is, the business end of the molecule. His breakthrough came in 1959 when he came across an enzyme, papain, which split immunoglobulins into three pieces, two of which were similar and could bind antigen, and the third of which had no binding ability but could be crystallized. The antigen-binding fragments are now known as Fab, and the crystallizable fraction as Fc.

FOUR CHAINS

While Porter was doggedly showing that immunoglobulins could be broken up into meaningful fractions, Edelman was trying the same trick, but in a different way, at the Rockefeller University in New York. With M. D. Poulik he treated immunoglobulin with chemicals that sever disulphide bonds (these are the links that hold the four chains together). Naturally, they found that the antibody split into two components, one large, the other small. The two Americans published their results in 1961, and what they said excited Porter so much that he wanted to try the experiments all over again to see what the relationship was between his fragments (from papain treatment) and Edelman's.

This he did, and saw more clearly what Edelman had shown before. It was then, in 1962, that Porter made the brilliant guess at the four-chain structure, which turned out to be right. From then on research on antibody structure roared away, with major contributions being made by Caesar

Milstein at Cambridge and Al Nisonoff at the University of Illinois.

The main obstacle to chemical analysis of antibodies was their extreme heterogeneity. If a batch of antibody taken from the blood of an animal contained a wide variety of immunoglobulin molecules, one would need some method for obtaining pure specimens of individual types of antibody; that would be difficult, time-consuming and tedious. At the time Edelman and his co-investigators had to know whether the antibody heterogeneity stemmed from many different ways of folding the protein chains of one single type of immunoglobulin, as was commonly believed at the time, or resulted from a wide variety of immunoglobulins with genuinely different amino acid sequences. If it was the latter—as was the case—the task of getting enough pure antibody of one type would be daunting indeed. Fortunately, Nature came to the rescue.

Occasionally one of the cells that manufacture antibody runs out of control; it becomes a cancer cell. In this condition, known as myeloma, the blood becomes flooded with lymphocytes and plasma cells all producing the same antibody. The blood of these patients is therefore a very rich source of comparatively pure antibody. Aided by this accident of Nature, and by Baruj Benacerraf, the eminent immunogeneticist, Edelman and his colleagues concluded that different immunoglobulins did have different amino acid sequences. This strengthened support for the selective theory of antibody formation. Remember, the template theory proposed that a single type of immunoglobulin was molded by incoming antigen.

THE FIRST ANTIBODY SEQUENCE

So, in 1965, armed with a knowledge of the four-chain arrangement, the Rockefeller lab set out to determine the complete amino acid sequence of a human immunoglobulin; they chose an IgG molecule. Four years of hard work, inspired by Edelman's drive and determination, brought the project to an exciting conclusion. At a scientific meeting held at Atlantic City in 1969 Edelman and his colleagues surprised the immunological world by announcing the complete amino acid sequence of a human IgG molecule. The Americans' brilliant success opened the way to confirming and extending ideas about immunoglobulin structure.

The variable and constant regions became apparent. More than that, the patterns of amino acids in the chains suggested that the molecule could be further subdivided. Edelman suggested the notion of domains (Figure 10), each of which was

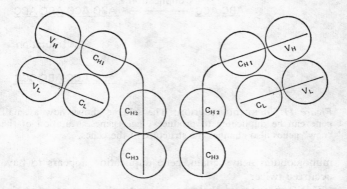

Figure 10. ANTIBODY MOLECULE DOMAINS: The antibody is arranged into specific regions (known as domains), each of which mediates a specific function (see text).

distinctly different from all the others, but they bore enough basic similarity to one another to suggest that they may have each evolved from a single ancestor protein. Immediately, this gave geneticists the idea that the genes for immunoglobulin molecules evolved from a single, much smaller gene. They argued that the original gene was probably big enough to code for about a hundred amino acids, that is, about half a light chain or a quarter of a heavy chain. Bigger genes

evolved simply by what is known as gene duplication; that
is, the small gene doubles up, thus producing a new one
twice its size. The new gene then further evolves by mutations
within the structure (Figure 11). In the case of the im-

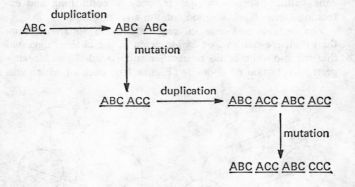

Figure 11. GENE DUPLICATION: The scheme shows how a small
gene can be duplicated to produce bigger genes. Mutation of the
"new" genes also changes the structure of the genes.

munoglobulin heavy chain, gene duplication appears to have
occurred twice.

Edelman suggests that these structurally discrete domains
evolved so as to separate the distinct functions of the antibody molecule. Structural separation of functional areas
diminishes possibilities of interference between the functions.
The variable domains are concerned with specific antigen
binding, while the rest have to do with effector activities.
C_H2, for instance, is important in complement fixation. C_H3
can bind to the surface of macrophages, something that may
be operative in arming macrophages and in mediating T
and B cell cooperation. In addition, C_H3 is probably also
important for binding the antibody molecule to the surface
of lymphocytes. Immunoglobulin molecules act as receptor
sites on lymphocytes, and the way the molecules are bound

to the membranes is almost certainly vital to the so far mysterious lymphocyte-triggering event that follows antigen binding.

THE BINDING SITE

The demonstration that the antigen-binding site is shaped from two variable regions of immunoglobulin chains went a long way to reassuring people of the ability of antibodies to create such a huge range of specific "locks" to fit the millions of antigen "keys." By having two protein chains contributing to the variability of the binding site the number of possible "locks" created is vastly increased. For instance, suppose there were just 1,000 different forms for the variable regions (there are in fact many more). With only one chain involved in the site the maximum number of possibilities is 1,000. But with two chains combining together the figure leaps to 1,000,000 (1,000 × 1,000). One can see how antibody diversity is achieved in terms of the protein molecules themselves. This again is comfort for the clonal selection theory, which demands that an animal must carry a vast range of lymphocytes capable of responding to millions of different antigens.

Genetics of Diversity

That, then, is antibody diversity at the level of the immunoglobulin as it appears after it has been manufactured. The next question about antibody diversity concerns the genes that specify the synthesis of this vast family of proteins. Both the heavy and light chains are probably produced as single protein chains carrying both the constant and variable regions. But evidence also indicates that, at some stage, the genes for the constant and variable regions are separate. For an immunoglobulin chain to be produced (heavy or light) separate constant and variable genes have to come together first. Edelman and one of his key collaborators, Joseph Gally, have devised a theory to explain how this occurs.

TRANSLOCATION THEORY

Their theory, known as the translocation theory, is that the genes come in three separate clusters: one deals with producing lambda light chains, another with kappa light chains and the last with all five major heavy chains. Within each of the three clusters the variable and constant genes are kept separate (Figure 12). The idea is that to make a

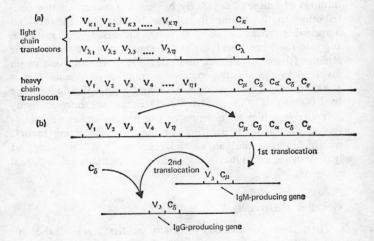

Figure 12. TRANSLOCONS: a. There are three main translocons: one each for the two types of light chain (lambda and kappa), and one for the heavy chains. Genes for the variable regions ($V_1 \ldots _n$) are clustered together, as are the genes for the constant (C) regions (there are five different constant regions in the heavy chain giving rise to the five antibody classes).

b. An antibody gene is made by a variable gene migrating (V_3 in this example) to pick up a gene for a heavy chain ($C\mu$); this forms an IgM antibody. The conversion to an IgG-producing gene occurs when the variable region then migrates again, this time attaching itself to a $C\delta$ gene.

complete gene coding for both a variable and constant region of the immunoglobulin chain, the particular variable gene is moved—translocated—from its original position and is inserted next to the appropriate constant gene (Figure 12b). Each cluster is called a translocon and is the basic unit for immunoglobulin evolution.

At some stage during the maturation of the lymphocyte the union of variable and constant genes for both light and heavy chains must occur so that when the cell is ready to go into action it is already committed to produce one particular type of antibody. How this happens, of course, is anybody's guess! Edelman and Gally's translocation theory provides a neat explanation for the way lymphocytes switch from IgM to IgG production during the primary response to antigen challenge. The variable gene is simply moved from a position next to the constant gene for a chain to a position next to a gene for a μ, γ chain (Figure 12b).

THE ORIGIN OF DIVERSITY

We have seen that the question of antibody diversity can be considered at two levels: the mechanism behind producing a vast range of antigen-binding sites; and the genetic machinery behind producing the required protein chains. Both of these are fairly well understood. But the third level of diversity—where the large range of genes come from in the first place—still remains perplexing. As we said earlier, there are two schools of thought: the "germ liners" and the "somatic mutationers."

The somatic mutation theory argues that all the variable genes exist in the germ cells that fuse to produce a new individual, that the blueprint for every antibody "lock" is present at conception. However, some people think a basic set of variable genes is handed down from parent to offspring, and this set is elaborated upon during lymphocyte maturation. Many immunologists (including Edelman and Gally) lean toward this latter view because of the vast array of genes that is needed to provide the observed antibody diversity, and because mechanisms for manipulating immunoglobulin genes —translocation—during lymphocyte maturation probably exist anyway. The two jobs might be done in similar ways.

Resolution of the germ line and somatic mutation theories is one of the major challenges in molecular immunology of the future. The other is discovering how a lymphocyte's antibody-producing machinery is switched on following contact with antigen. Edelman and his colleagues are now trying to find this out. They are examining the molecular architecture of the lymphocyte surface and are trying to discover the mode of interaction that exists between the receptor immunoglobulin and the surface membrane to which it is anchored.

One factor in the triggering mechanism must be the way that antigen is presented to the surface receptors on the lymphocyte. We will discuss this in the following chapter when we explore T and B cell cooperation—most recent revolution in a fast-moving science.

4. Cooperation and the Immune Response

Undoubtedly, 1973 was the year of the macrophage. The reason is that this unpretentious and long-neglected member of the white blood cell family is central to the fascinating and complex cooperation that operates between B and T lymphocytes. This cooperation, which is essential in almost all antibody production, represents another revolution that has transformed immunology within the last few years. The mechanisms by which cooperation is mediated are still the subject of heated dispute among immunologists the world over, but even though ideas about cooperation are relatively immature, they have already had profound effects on our understanding of important phenomena such as autoimmune diseases and cancer.

The Immune Response and Memory

Cooperation between T and B lymphocytes is at the heart of the immune system's response to a large group of pathogenic antigens which provoke antibody production. So far we have looked at the response from the point of view of the antibodies manufactured. Now we should examine the cellular events that underlie the response. Initially, we will ignore the T and B cell cooperation in order to avoid clouding the over-all picture with what in many cases are unresolved, albeit very important, details.

Animals carry about with them many thousands of different types of B lymphocytes, each of which is designed to recognize a specific antigen. The recognition sites are, of course, in the antibody molecules that are anchored to the surface of the cell; each B cell has between 50,000 and 100,000 antibody molecules scattered over the cell surface, each one capable of combining with the specific antigen to which the cell is "tuned."

In an animal that is virgin to a particular antigen (that is, it has not encountered the antigen before) there are very few of the corresponding lymphocytes. The essence of the immune response to the antigen is that as well as the production of a flood of antibodies to attack the antigen, the animal is geared up to respond much more rapidly to a second challenge by the same antigen. This immunological memory resides in an increased number of specific antibody-producing cells following exposure to antigen.

RESPONSE TO ANTIGEN BY B CELLS

When, in its surveillance activities, a B lymphocyte chances upon its corresponding antigen, the immune cell responds first by going into rapid multiplication: it starts to divide to produce more and more and more daughter cells. But the change is not just one of quantity; it is of quality too. Remember, the parent cell does not actively synthesize antibodies, except those that it displays on its surface as receptors. So the daughter cells must transform themselves into antibody factories. As the daughter cells mature, they begin synthesizing antibodies which are released into the blood. And as they mature still further they become transformed into plasma cells which are the real antibody factories, putting out many thousands of antibody molecules each second. Perhaps because of their total dedication and frenetic activity, plasma cells have a very limited life span of just two or three days. As the antibody-producing cells develop, they switch from panic button IgM synthesis to specific IgG.

Not all the daughter cells are destined to become antibody factories. Instead, some make no antibody at all and become memory cells. These cells are indistinguishable from the parent cell, except that the antibody receptors are usually

IgG rather than IgM, and there are more of them; in other words, they are already switched to the major specific antibody. Like the parent cell, they are sensitive to their particular antigen, to which they can respond by proliferating to generate plasma cells and more memory cells (Figure 13). The stimulus for continued creation of plasma cells and

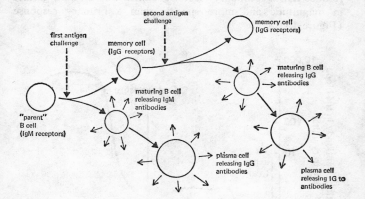

Figure 13. The formation of antibody-producing cells and memory cells on challenge with antibody. Memory cells tend to have IgG rather than IgM receptors.

memory cells is the presence of antigen. Once the antigen is mopped up the proliferation and maturation processes cease, the plasma cells die away and all that is left are the memory cells.

Once an animal has responded to a challenge by a particular antigen it is subsequently on the alert for a repeat challenge. Imagine a mouse virgin to, say, antigen A. Before it meets the antigen it has 20,000 B cells (that is, relatively few) lying in wait for the attack. Following a challenge, there are in the region of thirty times more memory cells produced than there were parent cells in the first place. (During an antibody response there are four times more plasma cells generated than memory cells.) Next time antigen

A enters the animal it is bound to run into a corresponding lymphocyte much sooner than happened in the virgin animal because there are so many more cells on the lookout for the antigen. Once stimulated, the memory cell can switch very quickly into producing IgG-manufacturing cells because the IgM to IgG step has already been completed. It is for these reasons that a secondary response is much more rapid, greater in magnitude and more specific than a primary response (Figure 14).

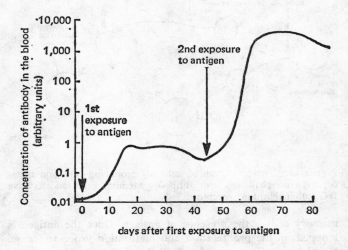

Figure 14. Antibody production in the primary and secondary response: Note that the speed and magnitude of the secondary response are much greater than in the primary response.

MEMORY AND IMMUNIZATION

Unlike plasma cells, memory cells can live for many months, and even years. The principle of active immunization —against smallpox and tuberculosis, for example—depends on the immunological memory mediated by the memory cells. If an immunized person never comes into contact with the disease organisms he has been protected against, the memory will eventually fade and he will have to be reimmunized to maintain his defenses. Usually, people are exposed to very low, subclinical doses of bacteria. Repeated exposure of this kind serves to jog the immunological memory by stimulating the sensitive memory cells; fresh memory cells are then produced to maintain the protection for several more years.

MACROPHAGES ARE RECRUITED

After an antigen has stimulated the production of antibody, that antibody recruits indirectly another population of white blood cells—macrophages—to help in the defense against the foreign invader. One effector function of antibody is to interact with a series of blood proteins known as the complement system. One result of this interaction is to punch holes in bacterial membranes. Another is to entice passing macrophages into the battle scene where they can devour the injured organisms.

Macrophages are a family of different types of related cells. Those that respond to the antibody/complement interaction are known as polymorphonuclear cells, or polymorphs for short. There is another type of macrophage, mononuclear cells (usually called monocytes), that do for T lymphocytes what polymorphs do for B cells, and we will now see how these operate.

THE T CELL RESPONSE

The basic T lymphocyte response to antigen is similar to the B cell's in that the T cell possesses surface receptors that can specifically recognize antigens. (There is a heated debate going on about the nature of the T cell receptor, and we shall come to that later.) But instead of producing antibody, T cells release lymphokines. These molecules, which are probably large proteins, attract monocytes into the area of infection so that they can digest invading bacteria which, meanwhile, have been attacked directly by T cells.

Antigen-provoked T cells therefore perform two functions: release of lymphokines to attract monocytes, and direct cell-to-cell attack on invading bacteria. (A third, and very important, function is to cooperate with B cells, but we will come to that later.) Like B cells, the very first response to antigen challenge is proliferation and maturation. And like B cells again, some proliferating T cells mature into memory cells that can respond to a second antigen challenge in the same way as the parent cell.

TWIN ARMS OF IMMUNITY

These then are the ways the twin arms of the body's immune defenses—the B cells and the T cells—react to invasion by foreign antigens. Apart from saying that one group of organisms (including pneumococci, certain bacilli, and meningococci) provokes a B cell response (humoral response) while another group (fungi, some bacilli, and viruses) provokes a T cell response (cell-mediated), it is not yet possible to describe in detailed molecular terms what determines which response will be activated. In practice there are relatively few occasions when an immune reaction to an antigen is exclusively humoral or cell-mediated. Usually there is a mixture of both responses, with one being perhaps more pronounced than the other.

This was the picture of the immune system's activities until just a few years ago. But the cooperation revolution, as it has been called, has shown how very much more sophisticated the whole operation is. Basically the "old" picture is correct. But as well as the considerable overlap between the B and T cell systems' response to common antigens, there is almost total dependence of B cell activity on T cells. Although the B lymphocytes actually make the antibodies, they cannot do it without the initial help of T cells. The discovery of cooperation shows T cells to be even more important than was thought hitherto, and the macrophage is seen to be a vital messenger in the immune system and not just a scavenger cell as it had long been dismissed.

Cooperation in Threes

No one disputes that cooperation exists in the immune response. But the mechanics of cooperation are not settled. Without doubt, research on the cooperative phenomena is the most active area of modern immunology, and will continue to be for some time to come. When a science is moving as fast and is as complex as cooperation appears to be, there are bound to be many running arguments and disputes among researchers. And when the scientists who are embroiled in the disputes are as outstanding as they are in immunology, one has a certain recipe for great excitement and immense promise.

The notion of the two immune systems working in parallel, sometimes overlapping, but being totally independent had great appeal. But a number of awkward observations made people begin to think that things were not quite so simple. For instance, immunologists discovered that if they removed the thymus from an experimental mammal they not only abolished the cell-mediated response, but also depressed the antibody response to antigen challenge. If the thymus, and therefore the T cells, had nothing to do with antibody production, why did its absence have any effect? Thymectomy in chickens also reduced antibody production. The absence of a bursa in mammals could therefore not explain the curious effect of thymectomy. The most paradoxical effect of all was that even when T cells and B cells were mixed together in a test tube they could generate only a weak response. Something had to be missing. It turned out to be the macrophage. People therefore began to realize that antibody production depended on B cells, T cells and macrophages—a cooperating trio. The question was, how?

EARLY MODELS OF COOPERATION

Avrion Mitchison and his colleagues, then at the National Institute for Medical Research in London, got some inkling of what was going on through some fascinating experiments performed at the end of the 1960s. They used small artificial antigenic determinants—haptens—which by themselves could not provoke an immune response: they were not immunogenic. However, if a hapten is attached to a big molecule such as the protein albumin it *will* be immunogenic. An animal can therefore be made sensitive to a particular hapten. But if the same hapten is then linked to a different protein carrier molecule and given to the sensitized animal the antibody response is much reduced. Why?

Some people attempted to explain this curious situation by saying that any individual lymphocyte had to recognize both antigenic determinants (the hapten and the carrier). But Mitchison demonstrated that a much more likely explanation was that both T and B cells were involved, one recognizing the hapten and the other the carrier. The British researchers then went on to show that T cells link up with carrier determinants and that B cells recognize hapten determinants. This idea led to one of the first models for B cell/T cell cooperation (Figure 15). The T cell first interacts with the carrier on a large antigen molecule, and then "presents" another determinant (the hapten-like portion) to a B cell, which responds by triggering the proliferation and maturation events.

THE CURRENT MODEL

The Mitchison model ignores the macrophage, which we now know to be vital to the cooperation phenomenon. Probably the best and most widely accepted current model—though by no means the only one—comes from Marc Feldman, who now works with Mitchison at University College, London.

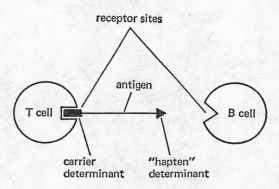

Figure 15. A SIMPLE MODEL OF COOPERATION: The T cell first interacts with the carrier determinant on the antigen; the hapten determinant is then presented to the receptors on the B cell.

The Feldman model involves an antigen message which goes from a T cell onto a macrophage and finally reaches a B cell (Figure 16). The sequence of events is this. Antigen entering the body reacts first with receptors on the T cell surface. The T lymphocyte responds by beginning to proliferate, during which time it starts manufacturing an antibody-like molecule which appears to be related to IgM. Unlike the IgM molecules manufactured by B cells which are arranged in fives (pentamers), the IgM-like molecule synthesized by T cells is a monomer.

The next stage is for the newly produced monomer IgMs to combine with antigen and then be released from the T cell. Now the macrophages come into action. When the IgM antibody/antigen complex comes into contact with a macrophage it slots into a receptor site on the macrophage surface. The macrophage has many such receptor sites scattered over its surface in the form of a lattice. Because the T cell IgM-like antibody now has antigen bound at the binding sites at the tips of the arms of the Y-shaped molecule the only part left with which to fit into a macrophage receptor is the stem of the Y, called the Fc part. After some time, therefore,

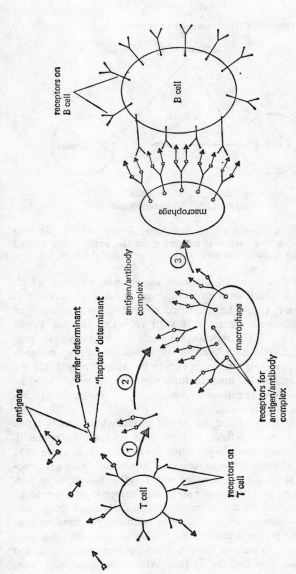

Figure 16. THE FELDMAN MODEL: Antigens attach themselves to antibody-like molecules on the surface of the T cell; the antigen/antibody complex then migrates to the surface of a macrophage where they are arranged in a lattice; the macrophage then presents the lattice of hapten determinants to immunoglobulin receptors on the surface of the B cell.

the macrophage surface becomes covered with antibody/
antigen complexes arranged in regular arrays and with the
antigen pointing upward.

The position of the antigen is obviously important because
the next step involves presenting the antigen to any specific B
cell that happens to be passing by. If the antigens bound to
the macrophage were buried or obscured, the receptors on
the B cell surface would not be able to react with them.
The final, vital event is for the B cell to be triggered into
proliferation and maturation. The way the macrophage presents the antigens to the lymphocyte is clearly fundamental
to the triggering process itself. Antigens that, when processed
by macrophages, can stimulate a B cell into action are unable
to do so if T cells and macrophages are excluded. Presumably, when free antigens interact with B cells they do so in
a random manner. But when they are presented on the
macrophage surface they are arranged in a neat lattice. It
is the lattice arrangement that is crucial.

In the middle of 1973 Feldman and another colleague at
University College, Mel Greaves, performed a neat experiment that supports the lattice idea. First of all they knew that
big antigens, such as large carbohydrate polymers, do not
need T cell cooperation. Presumably this is because the determinants are positioned as arrays on the natural molecule
and therefore do not need the help of the macrophage. Feldman and Greaves wanted to see if they could get around T
cell dependence for small antigens by arranging them in
artificial arrays. This they did by sticking a set of small antigens onto a microscopic bead, about the size of a macrophage.
It worked. The B cell triggered.

Lymphocyte triggering is just one of the many uncertain
areas in cooperation. In fact, Feldman's model at the moment
is no more than a good guess. It remains to be proved. But
supporting evidence continues to come from laboratories all
over the world. For instance, John Rhodes of the National
Institutes of Health in Bethesda reported in the middle of
1973 that he had found receptors on the surface of macrophages that would accommodate the Fc part of monomeric

IgM molecules. And early in 1974 a group of researchers at the Basel Institute for Immunology announced that they had shown T cells to be capable of synthesizing immunoglobulin-like molecules, possibly of the IgM class, thus fitting in with Feldman's ideas.

ANTIGEN COMPETITION

One very important and previously mysterious immunological phenomenon is explained by the involvement of macrophage messengers in the humoral response: that is, antigen competition. Immunologists knew that if an animal is being challenged with one antigen its response to a second, unrelated antigen is much less than one might have expected. Different B cells must be involved in the two responses, so why should the second be affected by the first? The answer is that there is a limited number of macrophages available to act as messengers between T and B cells.

Multifarious Macrophages

The family of white blood cells classified as macrophages has a major role to play in immune responses to antigens. Many of the more sophisticated roles of these little cells were discovered during 1973, a fact that led Leslie Brent, a former colleague of Sir Peter Medawar's, the famous British immunologist and Nobel Prize winner, to coin the phrase that "1973 was the year of the macrophage."

The roles of macrophages are many, and we should take a brief look at them collectively. First, macrophages can partially digest invading antigens so that lymphocytes can manage them more easily. When T cells react with antigens they prepare themselves to pass on an antibody/antigen complex for the macrophage to pick up as a passenger, as we have just seen. Earlier still in this chapter we saw that stimulated T cells release lymphokines, one of which, called macrophage-inhibiting factor (MIF), helps to localize phagocytic macrophages (that is, ones that can digest pathogenic organisms) in an infected area. (Incidentally, another probable function of lymphokines released by T cells is to amplify the antibody production of B cells. T cell cooperation therefore includes both triggering the antibody response and boosting it once started.)

MIF, or possibly an associated lymphokine, also incites macrophages into aggressive activity against any foreign cells that happen to get in the way; the macrophages are said to become "angry," a name given because of their furious activity seen under a microscope. B cells can stir macrophages into anti-bacterial activity by coating the invading cells with antibody. Macrophages themselves can bind antibody to their surface in order to make them specifically aggressive toward particular antigens; the antigen complex bound to the surface is known as specific macrophage arming factor.

As we saw earlier, there are several different types of macrophages: monocytes, usually associated with T cell activities; polymorphs, which mediate some of the B cell's effector functions; and granulocytes, the scavenger cells that form part of the first line of defense against bacterial invasion; the activity of granulocytes is much less specific than their cousins'.

So recent is the knowledge about the more sophisticated functions of some of the macrophages that immunologists do not yet know, for instance, whether the monocytes that become aggressive when armed with antibody are the same type of cell that takes part in cooperation. No one knows precisely how they respond to the various lymphokines and other factors aimed at them. One thing is certain though, there is a great deal more to be learned about these much neglected and much derided cells. Scavengers they may be, but they have great subtleties to their character too. Many biology books are going to have to be rewritten to take account of the new knowledge about macrophages.

Spin-off from Cooperation

The burst of research activity that the discovery of cooperation generated has thrown up a great number of important

issues concerning the immune response. Some of these we
have already discussed; others we should mention briefly
here. They are: the possibility of two GODs instead of one;
the role of cross-linking in triggering lymphocyte activity;
the suggestion of two types of T cell which cooperate with
each other; and the nature of the receptors on T cells. Like
much of current activity in immunology, a lot of what one
can say about these topics is inspired speculation rather than
proven fact.

HOW MANY GODS?

In an earlier chapter we discussed the problem of how the
human body can manufacture close to a million different
families of lymphocytes, each tuned to a specific antigen. As
we said, this generation of diversity—GOD—could either result from a genetic blueprint handed from parent to offspring,
or it may spring from a basic set of genes that become
modified during lymphocyte development (by somatic mutation, for example). It now seems that T cells and B cells
are very particular about the antigens they recognize: T cells
react with carrier determinants, while B cells bind determinants akin to the haptens of Mitchison's experiments. This discrimination makes good sense because if both types of
lymphocyte were attracted by exactly the same group of
antigens there would be competition rather than cooperation
between them. But how does the system work?

The most certain answer to that question is that no one
knows! But fascinating suggestions abound. For instance,
there may be two GODs, not one. One GOD produces one
set of specific antibodies (or antibody-like molecules) to react
with one set of antigens (carriers, for example), while a
second GOD leads to another entirely separate selection of
antibodies designed to bind with a different type of antigen:
in other words, one GOD for T cells, the other for B cells.

Carrier determinants and hapten-like determinants are
different in size: carriers are bigger. Mel Greaves of University
College, London, believes that a difference in size and spatial

conformation of antigens is more likely to be the basis of T and B cell discrimination than is a difference in molecular make-up, as the two GODs idea implies. Greaves admits that the answer might turn out to be a bit of both.

Another explanation rests on the tricky problem of triggering lymphocytes into activity. Many antigenic determinants can bind to lymphocyte receptors, but not all of them trigger the cell. There are probably a number of factors influencing the total response of a lymphocyte, one of which we will discuss in the next section. A particularly intriguing idea is that the ultimate activity of a lymphocyte may be governed by a special gene known as the immune response gene. This gene might determine which type of antigenic determinants would trigger, say, a T cell against a background of similar receptors in both B and T cells. Immune response genes might modulate the products of GOD, thus creating two separate populations of antigen receptors. But now we are getting deep into the realms of speculation. Undoubtedly, this is a fascinating problem and we will go into it in more detail in the next chapter.

THE IMMUNOGENIC TRIGGER

Antigenic determinants can bind to receptor molecules on lymphocytes, but they do not necessarily provoke an immune response. For instance, the B cell insists on having determinants presented to it in a regular array. This is not just to give the macrophage an interesting job to do. It must be basic to the molecular mechanisms behind triggering. And if the B cell is so particular about the way it receives antigens, what about the T cell?

The question of triggering comes down to a process known as cross-linking. All immunogenic antigens (protein molecules or large carbohydrate polymers, for example) have antigenic determinants repeated several times on the one molecule. This means that when such an antigen is presented to the surface of a B cell each determinant binds to an antigen-combining site on separate receptor molecules (Figure 16). In other words, a number of neighboring receptors are now linked together, hence the term "cross-linking." Unless neighboring receptors are linked together by antigenic detetminants the lymphocyte is switched off rather than on; it is said to be paralyzed.

When antigenic determinants are arranged in a lattice on a macrophage they are effectively a large, multi-determinant polymer. Cross-linking between B cell receptors is therefore assured. But just as too little cross-linking fails to trigger the B cell, so can too much. If antigen is present in a vast excess the B cell is once again switched off rather than on. The degree of cross-linking is critical. As we shall see later, this situation is important in inducing tolerance to particular antigens.

T cells do not need the help of macrophages to become activated. Stimulation of T cells requires cross-linking between surface receptors, but to a much smaller extent. Once again, the critical degree of linking between receptors probably plays an important role in establishing tolerance.

The triggering phenomenon is occupying the time of a number of very bright scientists. Gerry Edelman, for instance, is trying to probe the molecular events at the surface of the lymphocyte that are instrumental in spurring the cell into activity. James Watson, of double helix fame, is examining the processes going on inside the cell as it becomes either triggered or paralyzed. At the end of 1973 Watson and his colleagues at the Salk Institute in California claimed that these events involve the chemicals known as cyclic AMP and cyclic GMP. Antigens that paralyze a lymphocyte generate the synthesis of cyclic AMP within the cell; this chemical switches the cell off. Whereas, a lymphocyte presented with the required lattice of determinants synthesizes both cyclic AMP and cyclic GMP in a critical ratio; this chemical ratio stimulates the proliferation and maturation of the lymphocyte.

Cyclic AMP and GMP are now emerging as important chemical messengers in many vital growth processes within cells. Their discovery, particularly the relationship between them, represents one of the most exciting areas of activity in biochemistry. It is therefore particularly stimulating that two such fascinating areas of biology—triggering in immunology and growth control in biochemistry—should overlap in this way.

TWO TYPES OF T CELL

The discovery of cooperation focused attention on the activity of T cells. As often happens, the more a subject is studied, the more complex it turns out to be. Just so with T cells, for there are two different types, designated T_1 and T_2.

The discovery of these two distinct types of T cell emerged during 1973, and there is still a great deal of controversy about them. For instance, are they two entirely distinct populations of T cell, or are they related in that T_1 "matures" into T_2? The best bet appears to be the latter interpretation, and this is the one favored by Avrion Mitchison of University College, London.

What then is the difference between the two types? T_2 is the form that, when stimulated by antigen, develops into the mature T cell that cooperates with B cells or attacks invading organisms directly. (Incidentally, immunologists still do not know whether a matured T cell can both cooperate and attack bacteria. There may be two types with exclusive functions, or just one that can do both jobs.) The job of T_1 is to convert into T_2 when specific antigen approaches.

T_1 cells appear to be the basis of T cell memory. In a secondary response the great expansion of active T cells comes partly from existing T_2 cells, but mostly from the specific T, memory population.

Experimental evidence suggests that the conversion of T_1 cells to T_2 involves cooperation between the two types. When existing T_2 cells interact with antigen they potentiate the maturation process of T_1 to T_2 (Figure 17). T_2 cells may

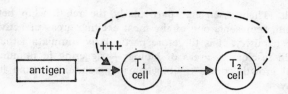

Figure 17. CONVERSION OF T_1 CELLS TO T_2: T_2 cells interact with antigen, and then perform two functions:
1) cooperate with B cells;
2) stimulate T_1 memory cells to mature into T_2 cells.

either help present antigen to T_1 or produce a soluble factor that stimulates the conversion. No one is sure about this yet, and it may turn out to be a mixture of both methods.

T Cell receptors

The receptors on the surface of B cells have posed no problem: there are between 50,000 and 100,000 antibody molecules embedded on the membrane with the fork of the Y sticking upward. These receptors are easy to detect with special biochemical techniques because there are lots of them and they are well exposed. But T cell receptors have proved recalcitrant to the desperate investigations of laboratories the world over, and they have generated one of the most intense disputes in immunology during 1973 and 1974.

The job of the T cell receptors is to recognize antigens. The molecules whose sole function in life is to do just that are antibodies. The obvious answer, and one that may prove correct in the end, is that T cell receptors are just like those on B cells. In 1970 Nancy Hogg and Mel Greaves in London were the first people to report the discovery of antibody-like molecules on T cells. A year later Jack Marchalonis and his group in Australia came up with the same suggestion. Since then about ten laboratories have got similar results, but many more have failed to find anything. For instance, Robert Good at the Sloan-Kettering Institute in New York claims that T cell receptors are definitely not immunoglobulin molecules; he has looked and he cannot find them. Good suggests that the recognition function of T cells resides in the pattern of molecules on the surface of lymphocytes, a pattern perhaps governed by the immune response given. On the other hand, a group of American researchers at the University of Wisconsin and the Wayne State School of Medicine, Royal Oak, Michigan, said at the end of 1973 that they can detect molecules on T cell surfaces that resemble partial immunoglobulin molecules which may have something to do with the elusive receptor.

One possibility is that if the receptors are indeed immunoglobulins there are very few of them—some people have suggested that there might be only several hundred—and they might be partially buried on the membrane structure. Other people propose that if T cells do have immunoglobulin receptors they may have imported them from B cells, a notion that makes cooperation even more complicated: T cells would need help from B cells before they could help the B cells! But at the beginning of 1974 a team of Swiss researchers reported good evidence indicating that T cells can manufacture their own immunoglobulins; they are not yet sure which class of antibody it is, but they are laying their bets on it being IgM. Furthermore, they say that the number of these antibodies on the cell surface is roughly the same as that on B cells, a fact that is very difficult to believe unless the molecules are so deeply embedded in the membrane as to be inaccessible to most techniques.

It therefore looks as if the logical and most attractive explanation—that T cell receptors are antibody-like molecules —is turning out to be true. But there is still the possibility that a product of an immune response gene could modify the antibody receptor, even if it does not constitute the whole receptor. Of this, more later.

Cellular Control of the Immune Response

We started this chapter by seeing how the immune response is switched on. Let us end it by looking at the ways it is turned off.

Immunologists have known for some years that antibodies can turn off their own synthesis. In the sequence of IgM to IgG production it is IgG that eventually brings the system to a halt. We saw earlier that IgM actually promotes its own manufacture; this is positive feedback. But when IgG production exceeds the amount of specific antigen in the local environment the excess IgG begins to inhibit its own synthesis; this is negative feedback. Excess antigen stimulates the system; excess IgG antibody turns it off. It now appears that these influences on antibody production are not the only ones. The lymphocytes themselves—particularly T cells—may play an important role in controlling antibody output from B lymphocytes and plasma cells.

The ideas on cellular control of the immune response come mainly from Leonard Herzenberg of Stanford University; Ethel Jacobson, who works at the Basel Institute for Immunology; and Anthony Allison, who is at the Clinical Research Centre, Harrow, near London. They find that T lymphocytes exert an inhibitory influence on antibody production, and that they act fairly late in the response. For instance, they discovered that if T lymphocytes are added to active B cells and plasma cells nurtured in culture, antibody synthesis is blocked. The inhibitory action is probably exerted by direct cell-to-cell contact between the T lymphocytes and plasma cells. It seems likely that the T cells involved in this control system are not the same as those that are sensitive to foreign antigens. It is possible, however, that these inhibitory cells may later mature into antigen-sensitive cells.

The question is, how do the T cells block the activity of B lymphocytes and their progeny? The answer depends on the fact that because antibodies are large protein molecules, they are therefore antigenic. In other words, one antibody can be

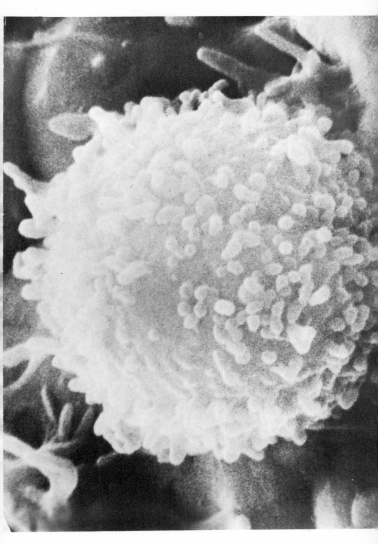

Under scanning electron microscopy, differences can be seen in human B and T lymphocytes that play a role in immune defense. B cells appear as complex spheres studded with large numbers of villi (finger-like projections). (*Memorial Sloan-Kettering Cancer Center*)

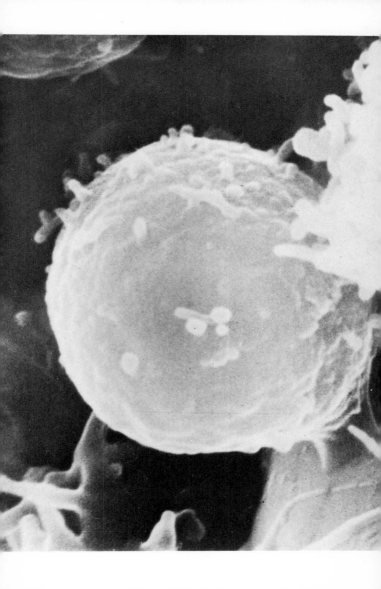

T cells are relatively smooth, with far fewer villi than B cells. (These cells measure approximately 0.005 mm in diameter). (*Memorial Sloan-Kettering Cancer Center*)

recognized by another because of the antigenic determinants on the molecule. In its turn the second antibody can be recognized by a third, and so on. A whole network of interrelated antibodies therefore exists, and it is on this that the fine control of antibody production rests. The antigenic determinants that are important in this control system are those displayed on the antibody's combining site; these determinants are known as idiotypes. It is this part of the molecule that is specific to that antibody.

A T cell that recognizes an idiotype on an antibody that is acting as a receptor on a B cell will suppress the activity of that B cell. In other words, for every population of specific B cells there is a population of specific T cells suppressing their activity, that is, stopping their reaction to foreign antigens. This inhibitory influence is counterbalanced because the B cell receptors also recognize idiotypes in other populations of antibodies. This recognition stimulates the B cells into activity. The upshot of the inhibition and the stimulation is a carefully balanced inactivity (Figure 18).

The balance of the lymphocyte network is disturbed when a foreign antigen enters the body and stimulates the population of B cells (via cooperation). This extra stimulation overcomes the inhibitory influence of the T cells, and the proliferation and maturation processes of the B cell population swing into action. As the foreign antigen is mopped up, antibody synthesis slows down and the whole system comes to a carefully controlled halt.

Antibody production should therefore be seen as a large series of interacting cell populations, some cooperating, some maturing and producing the antibodies, some stimulating and others inhibiting. The effects of invasion by foreign antigen therefore spread through a series of lymphocyte populations like ripples on a pond.

Scope for Controlled Intervention

Compared with scientists' view of immunity just a few years ago, current knowledge shows the immune system to be

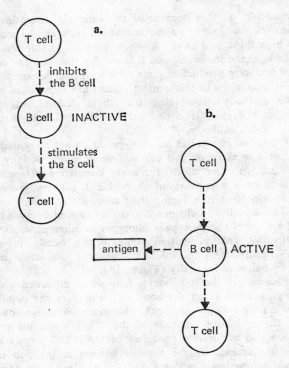

Figure 18.
a. The antibody-producing capacity of any particular B cell is kept in check by a network of inhibitory and stimulatory influences from other T and B cells.
b. When a foreign antigen intrudes, the over-all balance is disturbed and the restriction on antibody production released.

vastly more complicated. Instead of being dismayed by its newly revealed complexity (and there is certain to be more to come), we should be pleased. For the ultimate object of immunologists is to be able to modify the system's activity when it goes wrong or when disease—such as cancer and rheumatoid arthritis—sets in. The more subtle the system is, the more finely it will be able to be tuned by the scientists. As Mel Greaves says, "The great advantage of understanding the subtleties of immunity is that we can then be equally subtle in its modulation, controlling it without subjecting it to major abuse."

5. Genes, Disease and Immunity

Ultimately, the blueprint for every one of us is written in our genes. In common with the rest of the systems in our bodies, the over-all ability of the immune system depends on the messages contained in the genes. We saw in an earlier chapter, for instance, that the variety of antibodies we can manufacture is governed by the types of constant and variable immunoglobulin genes we can assemble. But current intense activity in immunogenetics centers on genes that have an over-all control of the immune response, independent of what antibodies we are programmed to make. It now seems likely that these genes—the immune response genes—may predetermine our susceptibility to particular diseases. A second set of genes that immunogeneticists are also keenly interested in are those that give us individual molecular fingerprints. These genes—the histocompatibility genes—occupy a great deal of the time of transplant surgeons because the products of these genes are responsible for initiating rejection of organ grafts.

A better understanding of immune response genes and histocompatibility genes is giving important insights into the mechanics of the immune system and will have a tremendous impact on clinical medicine.

Chromosomes and Genes

Every living cell in the human body contains forty-six chromosomes, apart from sperm (in males) and ova (in females), which have half that number. Chromosomes come in pairs, so in all we have twenty-three pairs, one of each pair coming from the father and the other from the mother. The chromosomes are made up of enormously long strands of DNA molecules linked together in a chain; packed around the DNA strand are countless thousands of protein molecules, many of which help to control the way in which the information in the chromosome is expressed. The information, which is eventually used to make protein molecules, is encoded in the particular sequence of DNA molecules in the strand. A stretch of chromosome six hundred DNA molecules long contains sufficient instructions to manufacture a protein molecule with two hundred amino acids joined together. Proteins vary in size, but each stretch of DNA chain that codes for one protein is known as a gene. Every chromosome has a DNA strand long enough to code for many thousands of different proteins—the chromosome has many thousands of genes.

Usually chromosomes contain one gene for one particular type of protein. Occasionally, an animal manufactures several different variants of the same protein, and they all do the same job. In this case there are as many different genes (or alleles) as there are protein variants. The possession of three or four protein variants is known as polymorphism, and it is not uncommon in Nature. What is uncommon is extensive polymorphism in which there are hundreds and perhaps thousands of protein variants. Polymorphism on this scale is seen only three times in vertebrate animals, on each occasion in connection with the immune system: the first concerns the huge collection of genes that produce the antibodies; the second, the unknown number of immune response genes that immunologists are just learning about; and the third, the histocompatibility genes that code for what are known as the major histocompatibility antigens. The immune response and histocompatibility genes are next to each other on one chromosome, while the immunoglobulin genes are located on a separate chromosome.

In this chapter we shall look at the way the immune response genes (Ir for short) were discovered and examine

some of the speculation about their role and how they perform it. And we will question why Nature thought it necessary
that we should each have a molecular fingerprint so that,
immunologically speaking, each person is distinguishable from
every other person in the world, unless of course they
happen to be identical twins. *individuality!*

Genetic Control of the Immune Response

By now it should be clear that the immune system operates
in anything but a simple and straightforward manner. With
three different types of cell involved, each interacting with
the others in intricate ways, the system is sophisticated indeed. It would seem a safe bet therefore that genetic control
of the system would be equally complex and that any geneticist tackling the job of sorting it out would be in for a very
difficult and frustrating time. As it turned out the task did
prove to be insurmountable for a very long time, but when
the answers started to emerge—beginning properly in the mid-
1960s—they were not as complex as one might have feared.

Evidence suggesting a genetic component that controlled
the immune response—whether an animal could launch an
immune reaction against a particular antigen—initially came
from two laboratories: Hugh McDevitt and John Humphrey
at the National Institute for Medical Research in London,
and Baruj Benacerraf and his colleagues at Harvard Medical
School. After staying in London for two years McDevitt, an
American, returned to Stanford University Medical School
in 1965, and since then he has shared with Benacerraf the
major responsibility for elucidating the function of the Ir
genes. When the breakthrough came for these people everything began to happen very quickly. Between 1965 and the
end of the decade they had opened up a whole area of immunogenetics which before had been buried in total obscurity
—five years is a short time in scientific research. By 1974 the
arguments had turned from whether genetic control existed
to how it operated. This latter question is proving to be one of

the most disputed topics in current immunology, and it promises to continue to be so for some time.

THE BEGINNINGS

The approach that finally cracked the seemingly intractable
problem of detecting a genetic control element in the immune
response involved using synthetic or semi-synthetic antigens:
the idea was to present an animal with antigens containing
only one or perhaps two different types of antigenic determinants. As we said earlier, a natural protein has many different
types of determinants on it; some of the determinants act as
carriers and others are a selection of different hapten-like
determinants. This means that normally an immune response
to a big protein involves the production of a number of
different antibodies, each aimed at a different class of determinant on the antigen molecule. In other words, the immune
response to such an antigen is very complicated and the
chances of dissecting out control mechanisms are minimal.
The idea of using a synthetic antigen with a very limited
number of different types of determinant on it is to try to
provoke a very simple immune response, involving perhaps
only one type of antibody. It is then possible to study the
genetic control of the production of that antibody in isola-
tion. This is what McDevitt and Humphrey and Benacerraf
did, but in slightly different ways.

When McDevitt joined Humphrey toward the middle of
the 1960s they wanted to look at the mechanisms of antibody
formation. They were using a synthetic compound called
(T,G)-A--L which is basically a long chain made up of lots
of molecules of the amino acid lysine joined together, with
side whiskers of another amino acid, alanine, sticking out all
along the chain, and with more amino acids, tyrosine and
glutamic acid, linked onto the end of the whiskers. This
curious-looking molecule is immunogenic. Or at least it
should be. But when Humphrey and McDevitt injected it into
their experimental rabbits they got very poor immune responses. Puzzled, they decided to try it on a genetically

different strain of rabbit. It worked. The first lot of animals consistently gave poor responses. Here then was a clear clue to some kind of genetic control of the immune response.

To try to get some clearer idea of what was going on the researchers switched their efforts to inbred mice strains. (Inbred animals are those that have been bred in such a way that as a group they share almost identical genetic make-up, just like identical twins. It is essential to use animals of a "known pedigree" when doing genetic experiments.) Humphrey and McDevitt gave their antigen to two types of mice, denoted CBA and C57. Although the CBA animals did not produce much antibody, the C57s generated lots. And when offspring produced by crossing CBAs and C57s were challenged with the antigen they responded much like the C57 parents; that is, they were good responders. The fact that two genetically different groups of mice reacted differently to the antigen—one was responders, the other was non-responders—strengthened the notion of genetic control of the response. The observation that the offspring from the cross between the two turned out to be responders indicates that the genetic influence for positive response is dominant, just as brown eyes are dominant to blue.

Humphrey and McDevitt continued their work by getting together a set of different synthetic antigens and giving them to the inbred mice. In some cases the CBAs were responders, in others the C57s were responders. So, having confirmed that genetic control was operating and that the gene or genes for responsiveness were dominant, the researchers set about answering a number of questions about the system: how many genes were operating, and did the gene or genes affect the structure or manufacture of antibodies? It turned out that for each antigen there was just one gene controlling the immune response, and that this gene had absolutely no influence on the actual manufacture of the antibody. In other words, the gene controlling the immune response was not the same as the gene that actually codes for the antibody molecule; the Ir gene appears to determine whether the antibody gene is switched on or off.

Meanwhile, Benacerraf had been doing parallel experiments
with synthetic antigens in guinea pigs. Using a hapten linked
to a chain of lysine molecules (to act as carrier), Benacerraf
also found that some groups of animals were responders while
others were non-responders. Again, responders were dominant. But the really intriguing experiments came when Benacerraf examined the animals' immune response to haptens
linked to different carriers. He discovered that what determined whether an animal responded was not which hapten it
was challenged with, but which carrier the hapten was attached to. Hapten A might provoke an antibody response
when it was given to an animal if it was linked to one carrier;
but if the same hapten was then given linked to a different
carrier the animal reacted as if it had never seen the hapten
before: it made no antibody (Figure 19).

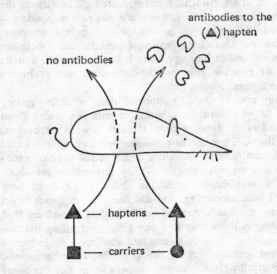

Figure 19. This mouse has no T cells that can react with the
carrier determinant on the left (■). It can, however, react to the
other carrier and can therefore initiate antibody production via
cooperation mechanisms.

These results imply that even if an animal has the potential to make a particular antibody, control of an immune response to the corresponding antigen depends on the ability to recognize the associated carrier. Interpreted in the light of what we know about the cellular cooperation in immunity, it seems that the immune response is controlled by the T cell system. That is, the Ir gene appears to make itself felt through the non-antibody-producing part of the cooperating trio (T cell: macrophage: B cell).

THE IMMUNE RESPONSE GENE PRODUCT

Genes code for proteins. So what protein do the Ir genes produce? No one knows. A lot of researchers would like to get their hands on it, but all they can do at the moment is infer what it is by what it appears to do. One interpretation of McDevitt's and Benacerraf's results—and the one that they favor—is that, because the gene appears to determine whether a T lymphocyte can respond to a particular carrier, the gene product must be the receptor on the surface of the T cell. We are therefore launched right back into the controversy about the nature of the T cell receptor. This is not an academic debate, because the immune response genes may prove to be a major influence on our health—whether we are susceptible to mild diseases such as measles, or are destined to die of a particular kind of cancer. We therefore need to know what these genes do.

So far attention about the target for the immune response gene has centered on the T cell. The most extreme view is that the gene product constitutes the T cell receptor and that it is structurally completely different from the antibody receptors on B cells. Against this view is the mounting evidence for the existence of immunoglobulins on the T cell surface. As we said earlier, there is increasing reason to believe that the immunoglobulin molecules that some people have detected on T cells are identical with or similar to the IgM class of antibody. Some researchers have already coined the label IgT for the T cell immunoglobulin if it turns out to be different from all known immunoglobulins. A number of immunologists believe that this T cell immunoglobulin is imported from B cells. But Georges Roelants' report from the Basel Institute for Immunology early in 1974 that T cells can make their own immunoglobulin seems to set that import idea back somewhat.

Even if the Ir gene product is not the major T cell receptor, there remains a good possibility that it could act as a second receptor alongside an immunoglobulin, or act to modify the affinity of the main receptor for incoming antigens. Another idea is that the gene works indirectly by controlling the number of receptors on the T cell. It might control the activity of other genes making immunoglobulin for the T cell, or it could influence the way the receptors are assembled into the cell membrane. Either way, numerical control of receptors could make a T cell either responsive to an antigen (if there were the right number of receptors) or non-responsive (if there were too few).

NEW IDEAS

Midway through 1974 the debate took a different turn. Until then the T cell had been almost unanimously elected as the prime site for Ir gene activity. But during 1973 and 1974 small strands of evidence began to appear suggesting that other cells in the immune system might be affected by the gene. To try to put these developments into perspective Marc Feldman, University College, London, collected them together and tried to weave a pattern suggesting possible alternative sites for gene activity.

First of all he pointed out that, using careful detection techniques, it is possible to see that non-responder T cells *do* have receptors for recognizing antigens, indicating that perhaps the reason for non-responsiveness lies elsewhere; in other words, T cells in non-responder animals might be perfectly normal. For instance, if the messenger macrophages did not have their specific sites ready for receiving the IgM antibody-antigen complex from the T cell the system would break down and the B cell would remain unstimulated. It is conceivable therefore that the gene product is a structural part of the macrophage receptor site. Alternatively, the gene product might be involved in the direct interaction between macrophage and B cell, again perhaps as some kind of surface receptor. Two pieces of evidence could make one sympathetic to this notion: first, the immune response genes are very closely related to genes that are known to code for cell surface proteins, as we shall see later; and second, a number of researchers are now getting hints that the B cells themselves are directly implicated in the expression of the gene product.

Another cell surface idea involves the newly discovered T cell/T cell cooperation. Remember that when antigen impinges on T cells, T_1 cells are converted into T_2. This conversion probably requires the cooperation of existing T_2 cells, possibly by direct cell-to-cell contact between the two types. The immune response gene could be important for the integrity of the receptor sites mediating this physical interaction between T_1 and T_2.

Lastly, it is possible that the gene is responsible for elaborating the non-specific soluble mediators (like lymphokines), known or unknown, that influence B cell activity in producing antibodies.

Once immunologists have sorted out this tangle, they will be in a position to contemplate modifying the system when it goes wrong, or manipulating it to enhance a patient's response to disease such as cancer.

AN EVOLUTIONARY ANCESTOR?

Hugh McDevitt recently posed an intriguing idea by suggesting the Ir gene to be a forerunner of classical antibodies in terms of evolution.

The structural analysis of antibodies indicates that, far back in evolutionary time, antibodies originated from a small gene about one quarter the size of the gene that now codes for the heavy chain. By doubling up twice, the small gene could give rise to a gene big enough to code for the heavy chain. McDevitt suggests—and it is no more than that, because ideas on evolution can never be proved—that as the small percursor gene evolved it first of all formed a primitive Ir gene that coded for immunoglobulin-like molecules that were always linked to cell membranes (the T cell's). The immunoglobulin genes (for heavy and light chains) might then have been established by families of the primitive Ir gene migrating out to other chromosomes where further necessary doubling up could take place. It's an interesting idea.

Clinical Implications of Ir Genes

By now more than thirty specific Ir genes have been discovered in mouse chromosomes. Some of these are thought to be associated with pathogenic conditions, particularly those involving susceptibility to viruses, such as Gross leukemia virus and lymphocytic choriomeningitis virus. For obvious reasons, mouse-type genetic experiments are not done in man and so there are no direct data on human Ir genes. But indirect indications are beginning to build up, suggesting a similar situation to that in mice; the number of putative disease-linked human Ir genes now runs into double figures.

Hodgkin's disease (cancer of the lymph nodes in the neck, thought by some scientists to be virally induced) and systemic lupus erythematosus (an autoimmune disease) are two important human diseases which are apparently genetically determined and might involve specific Ir genes. Unlike McDevitt's and Benacerraf's experiments with synthetic antigens, these two diseases are certain to present a very complicated antigenic challenge to the host and therefore the genetic control of the conditions would be very diverse and not easy to unravel.

In Hodgkin's disease it is conceivable that the immune recognition system (T cells, macrophages, or whatever) is deficient for the infective agent (possibly a virus) that causes the condition. An absent or a defective Ir gene could be responsible for the breakdown of the system. Because T cells are thought to be particularly important in detecting and destroying incipient cancers, Ir gene defects may play a very large part in determining which cancers individuals are susceptible to, or even fated to have.

An autoimmune disease occurs when the normally friendly immune system becomes aggressive and attacks the body's own tissues. Usually, one's own tissue antigens are tolerated by one's immune system (as we shall see in the following chapter), but occasionally the defenses turn hostile and we are attacked from within. Why this happens is still a matter of speculation, but it may be that the T cell cooperation is a screen against such overreactivity. When the screen breaks down antibodies against self-antigens may be manufactured. The genetic component in systemic lupus erythematosus suggests possible implication of an Ir gene in the disease.

The aim of many immunogeneticists is to confirm the existence of and characterize human Ir genes so that tests can be developed to see if specific ones are functioning normally. This goal is a long way off, but if it is ever achieved it will open up a whole new area of predictive medicine, and with it will come ethical problems too. For instance, a tiny drop of blood taken from a newborn infant could contain enough information to predict his medical future. And if the information written in the genes says that the individual is doomed to succumb to stomach cancer, Hodgkin's disease or lung cancer, what does the doctor do? Without methods for heading off such grim fates, there would be a great ethical dilemma about whether or not the individual should be told what lies ahead of him. Constantly surveying his anatomy for signs of the onset of cancer is likely to reduce "the patient" to a neurotic wreck.

Ir Genes and Histocompatibility Antigens

Almost all molecules are antigenic (though not necessarily immunogenic, remember). And because the membranes that form the outer boundary to each of the cells in our body are made up of many different types of molecule—protein, fats, carbohydrates, and mixtures of all three—the cell surface is covered with antigens. For this reason, when the tissues of one person are put into the body of another they are recognized as being foreign and are rejected by the immune defenses (unless the two individuals are identical twins or are very closely related). Not all the cell surface antigens are equally important in determining whether a tissue is recognized as foreign or not. The ones that exert most effect are known as the major histocompatibility antigens. It is these antigens that a transplant surgeon has to be very wary of when he performs an organ graft operation.

Geneticists have been probing the genes controlling histocompatibility antigens for almost fifty years now. The researchers were interested in the mechanisms of tumor transplantation and rejection. They soon discovered that there were no barriers to transplantation between animals of an inbred strain (who are genetically identical), but rejection always occurred when tissues were transplanted between genetically different strains. Systematic genetic analysis revealed that there were a number of genes, located on different chromosomes, that coded for the antigens responsible for rejection. It turned out that in man and in mice—possibly the two most intensively studied species—one of the genes was much more influential than the others: they are known as H-2 in mice and HL-A in man.

These major histocompatibility genes were soon discovered to be multiple sets rather than single genes—they are highly polymorphic, as we said at the beginning of the chapter. The major histocompatibility locus—as the collection of genes is known—in both mouse and man covers an area of chromosome capable of coding for perhaps two thousand genes. But geneticists discovered that the genes for the most important cell surface antigens are not spread evenly throughout this region; they are concentrated at either end, leaving a gap in the middle, possibly coding for many hundreds of genes. In mice the two gene clusters are denoted K and D (from left to right on a conventional gene map) and in man they are

Four and LA respectively. What then is lodged between the two clusters?

The answer came by sheer accident and "extreme good luck," as McDevitt puts it. For when Humphrey and McDevitt were studying animals' immune responsiveness and histocompatibility, they found it impossible to manipulate the histocompatibility genes without affecting the immune response. The implication was clear: the histocompatibility genes were linked to Ir genes (that is, on the same chromosome). As it turns out, the Ir genes are right in the middle of the histocompatibility locus; they fill the gap between the K and D clusters in mice and the Four and LA clusters in man (Figure 20). Incidentally, the fact that Ir genes are so closely asso-

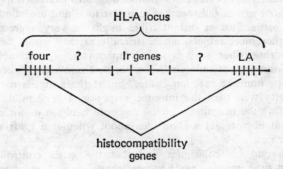

Figure 20. THE MAJOR HISTOCOMPATIBILITY LOCUS ON A HUMAN CHROMOSOME: The genes for the histocompatibility antigens are located at the two ends of the locus. In the middle are the sites for the proposed immune response (Ir) genes. There may also be other genes there which have to do with cell recognition.

ciated with genes that code for cell surface proteins was one of the initial reasons for thinking that the Ir gene product might be a receptor on the T cell surface.

The exact relationship between Ir genes and histocompatibility genes still remains to be established. Some people believe that they are simply different versions of the same gene, that they are in fact identical.

Tissue Typing and Transplantation

For an organ graft to survive in a new host it has to be anti-genetically similar to the host's tissues so that it is tolerated by the immune system. So before transplants are undertaken, doctors have to match up the donor's antigen pattern with the recipient's; in other words, they have to find someone whose molecular fingerprint is sufficiently similar to the ailing patient's. This matching process is known as tissue typing.

One of the most recent and successful techniques of tissue typing is that developed by Fritz Bach and his colleagues at the University of Wisconsin. The technique—known as the mixed lymphocyte culture (MLC) reaction—is simple and effective. Lymphocytes from the blood of prospective recipient and donor are mixed together in a test tube and are allowed to do battle. Just as distant tribes might be very aggressive when they meet rather than be friendly as they would be to neighboring tribes, so it is with lymphocytes: when lympho-cytes from antigenically dissimilar people are mixed a vigorous test tube immune reaction ensues, but if the antigens match up pretty well then the immune response is very mild. By measuring the magnitude of the response between donor and recipient doctors get a good idea about whether a graft will take or not.

Bach and his colleagues find that the genes controlling the test tube immune reaction are located in and around the H-2 region in mice and the HL-A locus in man. The fact that the histocompatibility genes, the Ir genes and the MLC genes are all located in the same area of the chromosome suggests that they may be a present-day version of what once was a primitive cell recognition system. The possibility remains too that Ir, histocompatibility and MLC genes are identical with each other.

Significance of Histocompatibility Genes

The two separate clusters of genes in the human histocom-patibility locus are responsible between them for at least twenty-eight different cell surface antigens. It is by juggling with these antigens, which are displayed on cell surfaces, that we each have an individual molecular fingerprint which is made up basically of four of the possible twenty-eight antigens. The most obvious effect of our molecular individuality is that there are great problems whenever a transplant operation is contemplated. It is conceivable that when Nature created histocompatibility antigens it was to make life harder for transplant surgeons. But it does seem unlikely, and more than a little perverse. So why do we have them?

AN AID TO EVOLUTION

Sir Frank Macfarlane Burnet, the Australian immunologist, claims that the properties of the histocompatibility antigen complex suggest that the system is important evolutionarily. The importance does not lie in the property of any particular antigen, but in that there is a wide *diversity* of antigens within the species. There appear to be sufficient variants of histocompatibility antigens to enable any individual of a vertebrate species to distinguish itself from any other. There are four main lines of evidence that support the notion that antigenic variability is important: first, every species so far studied has at least twenty definable antigens; second, there is good evidence to suggest that new antigenic variabilities arise relatively easily and that genetic mechanisms exist to assist the process; third, all histocompatibility antigens examined so far are located in cell membranes where they can be displayed as individuality "flags"; fourth, the similarity between the structure of the H-2 locus in mice and the HL-A locus in man is clearly no accident.

THREE IDEAS

So the virtue of histocompatibility antigens rests with their diversity. How does this help? In recent years there have been three major proposals on the biological value of the diversity.

TO GENERATE ANTIBODY DIVERSITY?

The first was from Niels Jerne of the Basel Institute for Immunology. He suggests that the range of antigens arose to help generate the immense antibody diversity we see in vertebrates. In other words, Jerne sees the antigens taking part in generating a somatic expansion of a basic set of antibody genes handed down from parent to offspring. The set of histocompatibility antigens in a developing fetus provides a "starting set" of antibody patterns upon which mutation and selection can act to build up the required diversity of antibodies: a testing ground on which antibodies against a wider range of antibodies are developed. But this theory may imply that the developing fetus has to "know" what antigens exist in other individuals of the species. And this implies, as Walter Bodmer of Oxford University says, "a parallel evolution at the population level of histocompatibility antigen genes and immunoglobulin variable-chain genes." This seems unlikely.

TO HELP COMPLEX DEVELOPMENT?

Bodmer himself proposed an alternative in 1972. He pointed out that for a multicellular animal to develop properly—to have all its organs and limbs of the right shape and in the correct place—the individual cells must operate some kind of recognition system: for cells to be able to sort themselves out in the correct order they must be able to "know" which cells are to do what. It may be, Bodmer suggests, that the polymorphism of histocompatibility antigens has developed as a consequence of the need to establish cell-to-cell recognition factors. But as Burnet pointed out at the end of 1973, the major histocompatibility antigens do not distinguish one cell from another, they serve to differentiate one individual animal from another. Moreover, the need for cell-to-cell recognition presumably is common to all complex organisms that undergo complicated development patterns during growth. That being so, it seems unusual that immunological function in the conventional sense is confined to vertebrates. If Bodmer were right, one might have expected polymorphism of histocompatibility antigens in invertebrates too.

TO PROTECT AGAINST INVASION?

Burnet's own idea first proposed earlier, but elaborated at the end of 1973, is that the diversity of histocompatibility antigens has been evolved in relation to the immune system to ensure that the body of one individual is not invaded by the cells of another from the same species. First, if there were no means by which one individual could recognize and destroy the cells of another, cancer would be contagious, a very undesirable state of affairs. Two other instances in which cells might pass from one individual to another are a type of pregnancy in which there is not a well-formed placenta separating mother from fetus, and parasitism of larger individuals by smaller ones of the same or related species. Both these situations occur in evolutionarily "primitive" species, and without the histocompatibility barrier, they represent potentially lethal situations, and ones that could be evolutionarily disastrous. Burnet calculates that all one needs to enable individual recognition is about twenty distinct antigens, a number very close to that actually observed in most species.

The trouble with evolutionarily based theories is that one cannot test them experimentally. But, as Burnet says, that applies to the theory of evolution itself.

This chapter has been concerned with the way one individual can reject the tissues of another. The next chapter is about the way we tolerate our own tissues, and what happens when tolerance breaks down.

6. Tolerance and Intolerance

The vertebrate immune system is remarkable both for the wide range of antigens it can specifically detect and destroy, and for the sophistication of the destructive mechanisms: invading bacteria, viruses and fungi are swiftly attacked and annihilated, and organ transplants are shrugged off with ease. In view of this constant vigilance and aggression, it seems a curious—but very desirable—quirk of the immune system that it does not react against one's own tissues. After all, one's own cells sport just as many potentially immunogenic antigens as does any invading bacterium or imposed organ graft. But the ability to distinguish between what is "self" and what is "non-self" (or foreign) is one of the three basic properties of the immune system and gives rise to the happy state of so-called self-tolerance in which—usually—we live in peaceful co-existence with potentially lethal weapons.

It was in the opening years of this century that, with his usual perceptiveness, the German scientist Paul Ehrlich drew attention to the phenomenon of self-tolerance. But it was not until the mid-1950s that any real progress was made in understanding the scientific mechanisms behind it. Australia's Sir Frank Macfarlane Burnet and Britian's Sir Peter Medawar were the two men most responsible for beginning to untangle the problems of tolerance, a feat that earned them joint shares in the Nobel Prize for Medicine in 1960. For more than a decade the concept of tolerance that flowed from the early experiments remained unchallenged. But now, with the dust from the recent T/B cooperation revolution beginning to settle, new and more precise ideas about tolerance are being proposed.

With them comes a better understanding of what goes wrong when the immune system suddenly starts treating self-antigens as foreigners and precipitates an autoimmune disease.

The Beginnings

Horror autotoxicus was the name coined by Ehrlich to describe the disastrous situation that might arise if the body's self-defenses turned hostile and set up a state of internal civil war. The problem of immunological tolerance and its apparent precariousness worried Ehrlich and he wrote extensively about it, but he did not get close to any answers. The first real clues had to wait until Burnet decided to switch from being a virologist to becoming an immunologist. That was in the late 1940s.

Like Ehrlich, Burnet was fascinated by the immune system's ability to distinguish between self and non-self and he felt that the phenomenon was fundamental to the whole area of antibody formation. Burnet has always been a great thinker, and it was thinking about two totally unrelated sets of observations that led him, with Frank Fenner, to propose the basis of tolerance. One observation involved virus-infected mice, and the other concerned non-identical twin cattle.

Many strains of mice are susceptible to a virus called lymphocytic choriomeningitis (LCM), virus which causes a form of meningitis. But some strains are not, and it turned out that these "resistant" animals had been infected with the virus via their mother's uterus, before they were born. LCM viruses in "resistant" mice grow well inside the animal's tissues, but they cause no disease; and the mice do not raise any antibodies against the viruses either—they produce no immune response.

The second observation that set Burnet off on his road to the 1960 Nobel Prize was made by an American geneticist, Ray Owen, working at Madison. Unlike humans, non-identical twin cattle (which derive from separate ova) share the same placenta inside their mother's uterus. Because the placenta deals with the blood flows of each twin, the blood cells from the two embryos occasionally mix. Owen noticed that after they are born each twin has a small number of blood cells from its sibling flowing round with its own cells. Normally such a cellular intrusion would provoke an immunological response. But in cattle it did not.

Here then were two potentially immunogenic situations (viruses in mice and blood cells in cattle) being tolerated. How? Burnet realized that they had one thing in common: in both cases the animals were exposed to antigen (LCM viruses or blood cells) before being born. Burnet and Fenner framed their ideas in a book published in 1949 in which they predicted that if any antigen was injected into an animal before its immune system had developed the animal would be tricked into treating the antigen as self and would forevermore tolerate it. Genuine self-antigens are tolerated for the same reason.

Burnet was in for one of the biggest disappointments of his career when he put his idea to the test. He injected killed microorganisms (as his antigen) into developing chick embryos. He predicted that when the chick grew up it would raise an immune response to every antigen except the ones in his microorganisms—it would be tolerant to these antigens. The experiment was a flop. After hatching, the chicks produced an immune response to the injected microorganisms just as they did to all other antigens that they had *not* been exposed to during embryonic existence. (Burnet realized much later that the experimental concept was right, but the technique was wrong. If he had given a series of injections of microorganisms into the developing embryos instead of just one he would have induced tolerance. It was all a question of too few injections!)

BRITISH EFFORTS

Meanwhile, British scientists were on to the same idea. In the early 1940s Peter Medawar, a young zoologist, wanted to do something for the war effort. So he turned his attention to skin grafting in severely burned patients. With a Scottish surgeon, Thomas Gibson, he learned that when strips of skin are taken from a donor and are grafted onto a patient they initially appear to "take," but very soon turn red and angry-looking; within a few days the grafts turn black and drop off. In contrast, skin transplanted from one part of a patient's body to another part heals perfectly.

Medawar decided that the rejection was basically an immunological reaction, and he set up a series of experiments on animals to test the hypothesis. He discovered that the rejection was mediated by immunologically activated lymphocytes (mainly T cells, as it turned out), and that if an animal is given two grafts in succession from the same source the second is rejected much more swiftly than the first. Here was a good experimental demonstration of immunological memory. But the major epoch-making experiment was done in the early 1950s with two colleagues, Rupert Billingham and Leslie Brent.

THE MAJOR EXPERIMENT

The experiment—which in 1953 was to create for the first time in the laboratory a state of immunological tolerance—involved transplanting skin grafts between different inbred strains of mice. The British team reared some pure-bred female mice and made them pregnant by males of the same inbred strain. Then, when the females were heavily pregnant, the researchers took a sample of cells from the spleen of a mouse of a different inbred strain and injected them using a very delicate technique into the pregnant female's uterus. The developing embryos were therefore exposed to the cells of a different strain of mouse. When they grew up the offspring accepted skin grafts from the second strain without the slightest immunological reaction—they were tolerant to the other strain's antigens (Figure 21). But just to prove that the animal's immune defenses had not been impaired generally, Medawar, Billingham and Brent demonstrated that the tolerized mice very readily rejected a skin graft from a third strain of mouse. The tolerization was specific for the antigens to which the embryos had been exposed during development.

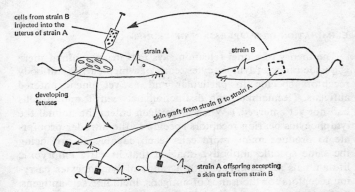

Figure 21. THE MEDAWAR, BILLINGHAM AND BRENT EXPERIMENT: Cells from strain B were injected into the uterus of pregnant mouse A. When the offspring were born they were given skin grafts from strain B. The grafts survived, demonstrating that tolerance had been induced in strain A.

Three years after this momentous experiment immunologists met in London, England, to thrash out a definition of tolerance. They decided that "immunological tolerance represented a specific central failure of the immune response to an antigen engendered by exposing an animal to that antigen when its immune system was still immature." This definition, which was very much along the lines predicted by Burnet and Fenner in their book in 1949, was well received for some time. But after a few years it became increasingly obvious that it was something of an oversimplification, as we shall soon see.

Clonal Selection and Tolerance

It is all very well to say that exposure of an animal to a particular antigen during its embryonic life induces tolerance specific to that antigen, but does not tell you how it happens. What appeared to offer the perfect explanation—and one that is still adhered to by some immunologists today—was the notion of clonal selection which came onto the scene in 1957, largely through the inspiration of Burnet.

ELIMINATION OR SUPPRESSION OF CLONES

The theory of clonal selection says that in any animal there is a wide range of lymphocytes, each of which carries antibody receptors specific to particular and as yet unencountered antigens. (Remember, the distinction between T and B cells had not yet emerged.) When an antigen enters the animal the lymphocytes bearing receptors specific to the intruder proliferate to produce many more cells, each capable of producing the same specific antibody. Imagine that in early embryonic life animals are equipped with a range of lymphocytes carrying receptors for thousands of antigens, including self-antigens. Self-tolerance can then be explained by suggesting that these potentially self-recognizing lymphocytes are eliminated or permanently inactivated. Acquired tolerance of the Medawar variety can be explained in the same way. In other words, if antigen encounters its specific clone of lymphocytes before the immune system is mature, those lymphocytes are destroyed (or suppressed) rather than stimulated. The notion is known as clonal elimination or clonal suppression.

FORBIDDEN CLONES

When he was developing his clonal selection theory, Burnet took account of the tolerance phenomenon and its breakdown. As well as postulating clonal elimination as a pathway to self-tolerance, he suggested that many self-antigens are kept permanently hidden from view of the immune surveillance systems: proteins inside cells, for instance, where T and B lymphocytes and antibodies cannot get at them. There is therefore no need for clonal elimination of lymphocytes specific for these so-called sequestered antigens because the immune system never encounters them. If, in adult life, one of these sequestered antigens leaked out and became exposed to the wandering lymphocytes, anti-self-antibodies (known as autoantibodies) could be produced. (As it turned out many of the antigens that Burnet thought were totally sequestered are present in the blood in low concentrations. Burnet did not know this because analytical techniques were not sensitive enough to detect them.) But the main mechanism by which autoantibodies would arise, he said, would be the generation of "forbidden clones." The idea here is that throughout life new clones of lymphocytes are generated (by some kind of continuous mutations) and that some of these clones would be self-reacting.

NEW IDEAS

Slightly modified, Burnet's ideas stood unchallenged for almost fifteen years, and for many people they still stand. But as immunological research gathered pace the flow of new evidence began to put clonal elimination and suppression in some difficulties. In 1971 two researchers—one in America, the other in Britain—independently proposed a new theory of tolerance, a theory that was made possible by the T/B cooperation revolution. (Remember, we now know that for B cells to produce antibody against a specific antigen, the antigen must *first* encounter a specific T cell which then presents the antigen to the B cell via a messenger macrophage.)

Two Kinds of Tolerance

The first cracks in the smooth façade of tolerance presented by Burnet and by the immunologists' London meeting in 1956 began to appear toward the mid-1960s. Two researchers in London—Avrion Mitchison and David Dresser—demonstrated that they could induce tolerance in adult animals, a discovery that went against the original definition which talked only in terms of young and prenatal animals. Not only that, Mitchison and Dresser showed that the specific inactivation of lymphocytes clearly is not as simple as Burnet's hypothesis might have implied, because they could induce tolerance in two different ways.

The experiments the British researchers did involved injecting mice with a protein, bovine serum albumin (BSA), which normally is immunogenic in these animals. But if BSA is given either in very low concentrations or at high levels the immune response is abolished. After low or high zone tolerance—as they are called—is induced, immunogenic doses of BSA no longer provoke antibody production. The tolerance was shown to be specific to BSA, confirming that the immune system was still intact. These results implied that there is nothing special about young, immature lymphocytes as far as tolerance induction is concerned, and that immunogenicity and tolerance induction probably involve more than one pathway.

With the increasing knowledge in the late 1960s and early 1970s about the duality of the immune system and the cooperation between the two types of cells (T and B), more precise explanations for Mitchison's results could be formulated. Immunologists learned that T cells are more sensitive to antigen than are B cells. An appealing hypothesis for high and low zone tolerance was therefore proposed which said that T cells are tolerized by low doses of antigen and that high doses inactivate B cells, and probably T cells too (Figure 22).

A number of research groups confirmed this idea by neat experiments on mice cells. They induced low zone tolerance in the animals by repeated injections of BSA. They then isolated the B cells from these animals and mixed them with normal non-tolerized T cells and exposed the mixture to an immunogenic dose of BSA. A perfectly normal antibody response was elicited. In other words, in the BSA-tolerant animals the B cells are perfectly capable of producing anti-BSA antibody, but do not because the T cells are inactivated, blocking the whole antibody response (Figure 22).

By similar types of cell transfer experiment, researchers showed that high zone tolerance involves both B and T cells inactivation (Figure 22).

Further doubts were cast on Burnet's original ideas when researchers found that they could experimentally induce antibody production against self-antigens that are normally tolerated. The experiments that revealed this phenome-

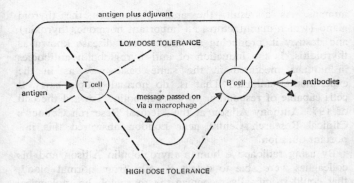

Figure 22. TWO LEVELS OF TOLERANCE: Normally an antigen provokes antibody production via cooperation between T and B cells (and macrophages). Tolerance can be induced with abnormally low levels of antigen (which blocks the T cells) or with abnormally high levels of antigen (which blocks both B and T cells). Adjuvants can bypass low zone tolerance by enabling antigens to react directly with B cells to induce antibody production.

non employed substances that are known to boost animals' immune responses; these substances, called adjuvants, are not antigenic themselves. When proteins from the thyroid gland (located in the neck), the testes or the brain are injected into animals together with adjuvant it is possible to raise specific antibodies against the proteins. Without the adjuvant, antibodies are not produced; they are normally tolerated. These proteins normally circulate in the blood at very low levels. They therefore seem to be good candidates for inducing low zone tolerance (that is, they block T cells).

The interpretation of these results therefore is that although the T cells specific to these proteins are inactivated, the B cells are still responsive (just like the mice with low zone tolerance to BSA). And because the adjuvants help the protein antigens circumvent the T cell cooperation stage, the B cells are stimulated directly to produce antibodies (Figure 22).

The thyroid protein used in these experiments—thyroglobulin—can in some cases invoke autoantibody production in humans. As a result, the antibodies attack the thyroid gland (which manufactures an important hormone, thyroxin) and destroy it, producing an autoimmune disease known as thyroiditis. Is the induction of anti-thyroglobulin antibodies in humans mediated in the same basic way as in the experimental animals? That is, do normal people carry B cells capable of responding to thyroglobulin? Toward the end of 1973 Anthony Allison at the Medical Research Council's Clinical Research Centre near London answered this important question.

By using radioactive human thyroglobulin Allison and his colleagues were able to detect B cells, from normal blood, that could specifically recognize the thyroglobulin molecules. These cells clearly have the potential to produce anti-thyroglobulin antibody; they do not because of low zone tolerance of the T cells. This indicates that thyroiditis might indeed be caused by bypassing the T cell cooperation stage. In contrast, Allison could not find B cells in human blood that could bind human serum albumin, one of the major blood proteins present in high concentration. High zone tolerance appears to be operating with serum albumin where both T and B cells are inactivated.

It was Allison and Bill Weigle, who works at the La Jolla Institute of Immunology in California, who independently proposed the new formulation for natural tolerance in 1971. They suggest that normal (or induced) tolerance results from a chronic reversible suppression of either T cells or B cells; antigens present in low concentrations (such as thyroglobulin) suppress the responsiveness of T cells, while high levels of antigen (such as serum albumin) inactivate both B cells and T cells. The major difference between this and Burnet's idea —apart from the distinction between two types of tolerance —is that Allison and Weigle see tolerance as a continuing suppression of immune activity rather than a once and for all inactivation. But the most important implication from the new ideas concerns the mechanisms of autoimmunity, as we shall see later.

The next question to ask is, how does suppression operate?

In an earlier chapter we saw that for a lymphocyte to be triggered a critical degree of cross-linking had to occur between the receptors on the cell surface; too little or too much antigen paralyzes the cell rather than activates it. Low zone tolerance probably represents paralysis of T cells because of too little antigen. To tolerize B cells in the presence of T cells appears to require an excess of antigen because an intermediate level of antigen might stimulate the T cells.

Evidence for two *different* mechanisms for T and B cell toleration comes from experiments on mice (in which high zone tolerance is induced, therefore tolerizing T and B cells). If a single large dose of human gamma globulin is given to mice, T cells become tolerant within two days, and remain so for a further hundred and twenty. On the other hand, B cells take between two and three weeks to become tolerant, and the effect remains for about fifty days. The fact that the onset of tolerance induction in B cells takes ten times longer to develop suggests that the molecular mechanisms involved are probably not the same. In other words, antigen excess and antigen deficiency probably provoke different responses at the cell membrane level.

Autoimmunity

Until very recently autoimmunity remained one of immunology's greatest mysteries. For although Burnet's proposal of the generation of forbidden clones sought to offer an explanation of the condition, many facts simply would not fit the story. Even though there is still a great deal to learn about this state of immunological civil war, the new information that has been flowing from immunology laboratories over the past couple of years now goes a very long way to supplying some long-sought-after answers.

TWO GROUPS OF AUTOIMMUNE DISEASES

An autoimmune disease is one in which pathological damage is inflicted on the body's tissues by specific anti-self antibodies. The diseases fall into two groups: one in which a single organ is affected, and the other where there is generalized damage.

Thyroiditis, sometimes called Hashimoto's disease after the Japanese doctor who first described it, is a good example of the first group. As we saw earlier, the disease arises when antibodies are generated against the very low levels of thyroglobulin that circulate in the blood. The antibodies progressively destroy the gland, eventually replacing it with fibrous tissue.

Two forms of anemia also fall into the first group of autoimmune diseases; they are hemolytic and pernicious anemia. In the former autoantibodies attack red blood cells directly and shorten their life from the normal 120 days to just a few days. The patient therefore suffers an acute shortage of red blood cells, whose role is to carry oxygen to all the parts of the body. Pernicious anemia is caused much more indirectly. Autoantibodies are raised against certain specialized cells in the stomach wall, destroy them, and thus prevent the formation of a substance known mysteriously as intrinsic factor. This factor is needed for the absorption from the stomach of one of the B vitamins, B_{12}. Without B_{12}, the body cannot make hemoglobin, the red protein that packs the inside of red blood cells.

The second group of autoimmune diseases is best exemplified by the disease we mentioned in an earlier chapter, systemic lupus erythematosus (SLE). Many tissues are damaged in SLE: skin, joints, stomach, intestine, spleen, lung, liver and, most of all, the kidneys. Unlike diseases in the first group, the damage in SLE is caused by a whole range of autoantibodies. And it is not a direct attack by the antibodies that inflicts the most damage; rather it is the irritating effect of antibody-antigen complexes that circulate in the blood and become deposited in the tissues. In the disease, antibodies to the person's own DNA and other constituents of cell nuclei are produced. Because the nuclei break up, antigens are released and these are then free to circulate in the blood combined with antibody. These complexes accumulate in the many thousands of minute tubes in the kidneys and literally block up the works: the kidneys aren't able to do their blood-purifying job properly.

Not all autoimmune diseases fit neatly into these categories. For instance, autoimmune hepatitis (a form of liver diesase) mainly affects the liver, but changes reminiscent to those of SLE also occur. Rheumatoid arthritis also has characteristics of both groups. The disease is thought to be caused by a curious double antibody complex (an IgG linked to an IgM). This "rheumatoid factor" circulates in the blood, but concentrates particularly in the lubricating apparatus of limbs. British research announced at the beginning of 1974 indicates that the immune complex induces the slow but steady release of harmful enzymes into the joints, resulting in the destruction of cartilage membranes there.

Causes of Autoimmunity

If one accepts the idea of Allison and Weigle, then the forbidden clone explanation of autoimmunity is untenable. The new idea of tolerance implies that autoimmunity arises when T cell cooperation is side-stepped. How might this happen?

If a tolerated hapten-equivalent antigenic determinant was linked to a new carrier molecule it would be able to induce antibody production. The new carrier would use a different set of T cells from the ones originally tolerized, and the B cells specific to the determinant could then readily be activated (Figure 23). One way this might come about is through virus infection. Virus-specific antigens are often seen in the membranes of infected host cells, and host antigens also become incorporated into the coat of virus particles. Viral antigens could act as a new carrier for the host antigen associated with it (Figure 23). A non-tolerized set of T cells would therefore carry the self-antigen to the waiting B cells. There is a growing body of evidence of autoantibodies associated with virus infections: for instance, as infectious mononucleosis infection passes off a selection of autoanti-

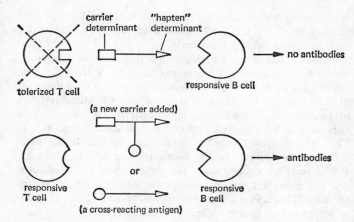

Figure 23. MECHANISMS OF AUTOIMMUNITY: In the first case the hapten determinant cannot induce antibody formation because the T cell corresponding to the carrier determinant on the antigen is tolerized (as in low zone self-tolerance). But if a new carrier is added or the hapten detaches itself from the old carrier and links up with a new carrier antibody production can be initiated.

bodies can often be detected; human virus infections such as influenza, measles, varicella, Coxsackie and herpes simplex often leave a trail of autoantibodies behind them.

A second possible mechanism involves a phenomenon known as cross-reaction. If two different antigens contain determinants some of which are structurally similar to each other, they may elicit the same antibody; that is, they activate the same B cell. But because the rest of the antigen molecule is different, different T cell systems are employed. Now, suppose a foreign antigen entered the body carrying a number of determinants in common with some self-antigens. Normally, the self-antigen would be tolerated because of low zone tolerance via a specific T cell population. But the intruding antigen can now stimulate the specific autoantibody formation because it activates a different T cell group (Figure 23). Researchers have demonstrated that a group of streptococci share common antigens with human heart tissue. And autoantibody production has been provoked in many experimental situations by infecting animals with different types of microorganisms. A number of autoimmune diseases probably arise in this way.

One marked feature of autoimmune diseases is that they run in families; there must therefore be some form of genetic component. As we saw in the previous chapter, one possible explanation is that a defective immune response gene either allows an increased susceptibility to infection by viruses or other organisms, or may result in an overresponsive specific population of lymphocytes.

T Cell Suppression of Autoimmunity

Self-tolerance seems to be so precariously balanced that it is desirable to have an additional protection. The recent novel idea of suppression of antibody production by direct (or possibly indirect) action of T cells on B cells fulfills this role nicely. (Remember, some T cells recognize specific antibodies on the surface of B cells, and by so doing, keep the B cells switched off.) In an earlier chapter we saw how control of B cell activity by T cells was probably part of a larger system of checks and balances governing antibody production. It could be that these controlling T cells also perform a sort of surveillance function, roaming the body on the lookout for the forbidden activity of anti-self B lymphocytes. If the surveillance breaks down a delicately balanced anti-self B cell may swing into action and produce autoantibodies.

One line of evidence in favor of this idea comes from a strain of mouse—NZB—that is particularly prone to autoimmune diseases. One reason for this is that their T cells are very difficult to tolerize; that is, low zone tolerance cannot occur properly. But a second reason may be that, because their T cell function declines rapidly as they grow older, the T cell surveillance system collapses and clones of anti-self lymphocytes become active.

Aging and Autoimmunity

There are many theories about why animals age (wear out and die), but no one can claim to have the answer. One of these theories—promulgated both by Burnet and particularly by Roy Walford at the University of California School of Medicine—concerns changes in the immune system as animals get older. Specifically, the "pure" immunological theory of aging states that the cause lies with built-in increase in autoantibody production as animals get older. The tissue damage thus caused is responsible, the theory claims, for the observed decline in physiological function with increasing age.

There does appear to be some increase in the appearance of autoantibodies as people get older, but this apparent progression is by no means universally accepted. Probably the strongest piece of evidence in favor of an immunological cause of aging is the curious life history of the thymus gland, the gland responsible for processing mature T lymphocytes. In humans, the thymus is at its biggest size relative to the rest of the body immediately at birth. It continues growing, of course, but not as fast as other organs in the body. It peaks at its absolute maximum size at six to eight years of age. From the age of twenty to twenty-five it begins to decline until only remnants of its outer tissue remain by fifty years of age.

Because the thymus disappears in this dramatic way, the competence of the immune system probably suffers. For instance, if there is a fall in the number of T cells that control B cell function, there could be a rise in the activity of anti-self lymphocytes, giving a rise in autoantibodies which could inflict general damage. Furthermore, there appears to be a rise in the incidence of cancer with increasing age. And since one of the T cell functions is thought to be as a surveillance system for incipient cancers, this rise could be interpreted as a sign of immunological decline. But old people are known to reject organ grafts much more vigorously than one might have expected if the disappearance of the thymus really does signal the end of T cell competence. The answer may be that, because T cells have a life span of many years in the circulation system, the absence of newly generated T cells may be of no consequence as far as normal T cell functions are concerned.

After a period of popularity some years ago, the immunological theory of aging is itself on the decline.

7. Cancer and Transplants

As far as immunologists are concerned, cancer and organ transplants are closely related: scientists would like to encourage our bodies to accept one (transplants), while rejecting the other (cancer). Doctors' efforts in preventing rejection of transplanted organs have given the immunologists important clues about the relationship between cancer and the immune response. And immunology could develop into the doctors' major weapon against cancer in the 1970s.

Cancer, the Enemy Within

First, what is cancer? Although scientists can describe what it does, no one yet knows exactly how it arises, beyond saying that viruses and chemicals are often involved. Perhaps the most obvious property of cells that have been made cancerous is that they stop obeying the normal rules of the body. For instance, instead of growing and dividing slowly and in a controlled way, their growth becomes wild and uncontrolled—they do not obey the stop signal as other cells do. This uncontrolled proliferation makes cancer a fatal disease.

In recent years scientists have discovered that one of the main molecular differences between normal and cancer cells shows up in the cell membrane. The chemical composition of the cell surface changes slightly when a cell is transformed, and the molecular patterns—the spatial arrangement of molecules—on the membrane alter too. Because it is via the messages sketched in the membrane's molecular patterns that cells communicate with each other, it is not surprising that cancer cells fail to respond properly to normal intercellular instructions.

Another consequence of the membrane modifications in cancer cells is that the antigenic picture they present is often foreign to the host. It is upon this assumed foreignness that an effective immune reaction to cancer must depend. In this chapter we shall see how effective the immune defenses against cancer really are, and why, under some circumstances, the aberrant cells escape and win the battle. We shall see too what immunologists are doing to try to make the immune system our most effective defense—and even prevention—against cancer.

Evidence for an Immune Response to Cancer

In 1973 half a million Americans died of cancer. Cancer is responsible for 20 per cent of all deaths in the Western world. The disease can therefore claim to be very prevalent by any standards. Yet the number of clinical cases of cancer that doctors see is only a tiny fraction of the incipient cancers that arise in our bodies. Probably thirty-nine out of forty times the cancer threat simply goes away or is destroyed; it is the fortieth threat that wins through and becomes manifest as a clinical cancer.

These figures—of a one in forty chance of incipient cancers developing—come from post-mortem examinations of people who have died from causes other than cancer. Doctors find a forty times greater incidence of cancers in, say, road accident victims than in the general population. The fact that the vast majority of new cancers do not become clinically established implies that our body has a pretty efficient system to cope with the threat, most of the time. Even with fully established cancers there are many examples of spontaneous disappearance of the growth. Immunologists have noticed that many of these spontaneous regressions coincided with some kind of bacterial infection in the patient—it looked as if the infection might even be responsible for the cancer's disappearance, perhaps due to cross-reactivity between the bacterial and cancer antigens.

So what is this anti-cancer weapon that prevents the disease taking hold and that might even launch a successful attack when the cancer has escaped through the protective net? There is now overwhelming evidence that defense against cancer is one of the many important jobs carried out by the immune system. The evidence comes from clinical observations, from clinical manipulations and from experiments with laboratory animals.

IMMUNODEFICIENCY DISEASES AND CANCER

For instance, doctors and researchers who deal with people suffering from immunodeficiency diseases—where the immune system fails to work properly—observe that their patients are more than ten times more likely to develop cancer than people whose immune defenses are intact. This suggests that a normal immune response acts as a barrier to malignancy (cancer). Robert Good, director of the Memorial Sloan-Kettering Cancer Center in New York, goes so far as to say that in every case of cancer he has seen the immune system has been screwed up in some way. Quite possibly, the immune response is blunted when a cancer takes hold, so that Good is observing a result of cancer, not its cause. But the lessons from immunodeficient patients make one sympathetic to the notion that specific immunodeficiency (a defective Ir gene perhaps) in apparently normal people could be an important contributory factor in many cancers.

ORGAN TRANSPLANTS AND CANCER

Experiences with organ transplants also reinforce the idea of an anti-cancer role for immunity. As we saw earlier, only identical twins have tissues that are totally acceptable to each other's immune systems. In most cases doctors have to damp down the immune response in a patient receiving an organ graft. After the early clinical trials of kidney transplants had been going for some time (they started in the early 1960s) it became apparent that some of the transplanted kidneys contained tiny undetected cancer foci. As soon as the kidney was put into the immunosuppressed patient the cancer began to flourish. This happened in nine cases, and in four of them the cancer rapidly spread throughout the body. Somewhat alarmed, the doctors realized that all they had to do was halt the immunosuppressive therapy. In most cases the cancer deposits disappeared with remarkable speed.

As kidney transplants became established, and more and more lives were saved, data were built up on the incidence of cancers in these patients after their operations. The prevalence of cancer in these people is ten times higher than in the general population. Once again, this was attributed to the immunosuppression that the patients were subjected to so that the new organ would be accepted. If the immune system is prevented from doing its job new cancers become established more frequently.

CANCER IN MICE

Lastly, studies on experimentally induced cancers in mice confirm the immune system's role in cancer control. It is possible to immunize a mouse, say, against a particular cancer so that any subsequent challenges with the cancer are shrugged off. The technique is to induce a cancer in the animal and then remove the tumor surgically soon after it is established. Any attempt to implant cells of the same cancer into the animal fails because of a vigorous immune response. Clearly, in this case the immune system can recognize cancer tissue as being foreign and can build up a normal immunological memory against it.

Cancer Antigens

For the immune system to be able to recognize cancer cells as being foreign those cells must be flying foreign flags in the form of non-self-antigens. The study of cancer antigens

—usually called tumor antigens—is presenting researchers with very sticky problems at the moment. What the scientists want to know is, do cancers have antigens specific to themselves, and if so, what controls them? With a better knowledge of what makes cancer cells different from normal cells, immunologists will be able to contemplate manipulating the immune response to attack those cancers that become established.

In animals—and possibly in man too—viruses and chemicals are two important causes of cancers. The antigenic picture of a virally induced cancer is different from one caused by chemical carcinogens. Current research on animal cancers concerns the individuality of cancer antigens and how far they may be important in invoking an immune reaction.

CHEMICALLY INDUCED CANCER IN ANIMALS

Chemically induced cancers in animals display two types of tumor antigen. The first is characteristic of a particular cancer in a particular animal. If a carcinogen—usually a chemical called methylcholanthrene—produces a muscle tumor in animal A the new cancer antigen that appears will be different from the new antigen produced on a methylcholanthrene-induced muscle tumor in animal B. The antigens are said to be not cross-reacting: an antibody to one of the antigens will not recognize the antigen on the other tumor. This class of chemically induced tumor antigens is so erratic that if two cancers are induced in different tissues in the same animal, the new antigens will almost certainly be distinct; they will not cross-react.

The second class of chemically induced tumor antigens is cross-reactive. This means that if antibodies are raised against the antigens on a tumor in one animal, the antibodies will react with the antigens on a similar tumor in a second animal of the same species. (The question of cross-reactivity is very important to immunologists because unless muscle cancers, for instance, share the same antigens, it is going to be very difficult to devise a rational large-scale immuno-

logical treatment of cancers. If every cancer has its own
non-cross-reacting antigen, each case will have to be treated
individually, and the prospects for vaccinating against cancers
arising would be non-existent.) Some of these cross-reacting antigens belong to a class of fetal antigens, about which
we shall learn more later.

VIRALLY INDUCED CANCER IN ANIMALS

In contrast to chemically induced cancer antigens, those
on virally induced tumors always cross-react. This is because
when the virus enters the cell, it makes use of the cell's
protein synthesizing machinery to translate some of the information in the viral genetic material. The new viral protein
that is formed finds its way to the surface of the cell's outer
membrane, where it displays itself as an antigen specific
to the invading virus. So, any cell that is infected by a
particular type of virus always has the same antigen on its
membrane; hence the cross-reactivity between specific virally
induced tumors. Compare this with a chemically induced
tumor in which the new antigens are generated when the
carcinogen interferes in a semi-random way with the invaded
cell's normal genetic machinery; the nature of the new antigen
depends on which particular part of the machinery is damaged.

The transformation of a normal cell into a cancer cell
is a complex process and the antigenic changes overall are
certain to be more diverse than implied here. The immunologists cannot hope to be able yet to untangle the
complexity of the changes, and at the moment they are con-
centrating on the ones that are most predictable and may
possibly be exploitable for clinical ends. So far, the cancer
antigens offering most hope of clinical exploitation are those
associated with viruses.

ONCOFETAL ANTIGENS

In addition to the tumor antigens arising from viral proteins (in virally induced tumors) and modified cell proteins

(in chemically induced tumors), there is sometimes a third set of antigens (arising in either chemically or virally induced tumors): these are the fetal antigens. During embryonic development there appear to be a number of molecular flags on the maturing cell surfaces which probably help in intercellular signaling. These molecular flags are known as fetal antigens. When the animal has fully developed, the flags are no longer required so the cells stop producing them; those in the membrane disappear. Normal cells in a fully developed animal (at birth) therefore do not carry fetal antigens; the genes that code for the fetal antigens are said to be switched off. Occasionally, when a cell is transformed into a cancer cell these genes are switched on again, opening the way for fetal antigen production.

Fetal antigens in cancer cells—sometimes known inelegantly as oncofetal antigens—come in two classes: those that are readily released into the circulation, and others that remain bound to the cancer cell surface. Immunologists do not know yet whether the cell-bound antigens are important in the immune response to cancers in humans, but there are some experiments on animals that suggest they might be. The antigens released into the blood almost certainly are not. But what these soluble antigens might be useful for is diagnosing cancer, as we shall see later.

HUMAN ANTIGENS

The big story concerning human cancer antigens began in Sweden in the mid-1960s. Husband-and-wife team Karl and Ingegerd Hellström discovered that if they took cancer cells from a patient, put them in a test tube and added the patient's own lymphocytes (after washing them) to the same test tube, the cancer cells were destroyed. This was a clear demonstration that cancer patients possess lymphocytes capable of destroying their own tumors. The Hellströms then moved to the University of Washington, Seattle, where they pursued the story.

The Hellströms went on to discover that not only could

the lymphocytes from a patient with, say, skin cancer destroy his own tumor, but they could kill any human skin cancer. But if the lymphocytes from a patient with skin cancer are mixed with cells from, say, human liver cancer there is no effect. Clearly, there are antigens on human cancer cells that cross-react between individual patients. Lymphocytes in cancer patients are specifically tuned to a particular type of antigen characteristic of a certain class of tumor (skin, liver, nervous system, for example).

Why, then, don't these lymphocytes attack the cancer in the patient? The answer is that there is some kind of blocking factor in the blood that stops the lymphocytes from getting at the cancer cells. We shall hear more about this later in this chapter when we discuss the ways cancer cells escape through the surveillance network.

The great problem with human cancer antigens is knowing whether they are immunologically significant: can the immune system make use of them to attack the internal intruder? As the Hellström's results foretold, human cancer antigens are turning out to show greater cross-reactivity than many animal cancer antigens. As we saw earlier, cross-reactivity is an encouraging sign in terms of developing therapeutic techniques. But although many human cancer antigens show immunogenicity and cross-reactivity in test tube experiments, when they are in people many cancers appear to be only very weakly antigenic, a fact that is causing immunologists a great many headaches.

Immunological Surveillance

In the mid-1950s Lewis Thomas, then at the University of Minnesota but now president of the Memorial Sloan-Kettering Cancer Center, was pondering why advanced animals should have such an efficient mechanism for rejecting transplants. Not simply to confound the transplant surgeon, he thought. Maybe it was to protect the animal from invasion of foreign tissue arising spontaneously from within; in other words, to maintain a constant lookout for cancer. At the time he was working with Robert Good on immunodeficiency, and in 1958 he predicted that if his idea was correct, their immunodeficient patients "would have too much cancer" because their surveillance system was operating at half cock. He was right, of course. Subsequently, this notion was elaborated and popularized by Burnet and it became generally known as immunological surveillance.

Robert Good believes that, far from being just one of the functions of cell-mediated immunity (carried out by the T cells), surveillance for incipient cancers was probably the reason that the whole system was evolved in the first place. As more advanced creatures evolved from their primitive ancestors, animals became more and more complex structurally. This meant that in these more complex animals the rapid growth and interactions between the specialized groups of tissues offered more opportunities for mutant cells to arise. If they were not kept in check these mutant cells might overrun and destroy the unfortunate animal. Good suggests that to combat this danger animals evolved a system to distinguish between self and non-self—the immune system. In Good's argument—which is not universally accepted— immunological surveillance is the most basic and primitive role of the immune system.

The surveillance concept was attractive and it gathered a great deal of support among immunologists, but there are some disbelievers. For instance, toward the end of 1973 Peter Alexander of the Chester Beatty Research Institute, London, said that "immunological surveillance is a name in search of a function." His view may be a little extreme, but it is now becoming clear that the surveillance concept is not as straightforward as was originally envisaged. As initially constructed, immunological surveillance would have predicted that in the absence of immunological competence (during immunosuppression, for instance) a general rise in the incidence of all types of cancers would result. But although there is a rise in cancer incidence in immunosuppressed patients, the cancers are largely of the lymphoid system, that is, the tissues of the immune system itself. A similar picture is seen in immunodeficient patients.

The cancers are by no means totally confined to lymphoid tissues—there is a rise in cancers of other organs too—but the variety of organs affected and the magnitude of the effect are not as great as one would have expected if immunological surveillance were responsible for combating all cancers. One possibility is that the cancers that escape when the immunological defenses are lowered are those with a common origin—cancers of the lymphoid tissues may, for instance, all be caused by viruses. To support this idea one can say that human leukemia is one of the prime candidates for a viral etiology. And Burkitt's lymphoma (cancer of one of the lymph glands in the face) has had a long history of viral association, but a causal relationship has yet to be proved. A predilection of immunological surveillance activity for virally induced cancers may simply reflect the greater antigenicity of these types of cancers.

Immunological Weapons Against Cancer

Until very recently, the anti-cancer picture was very simple for immunologists: T cells were good at combating cancer, but B cells were bad at it, not just because they could not kill cancer cells, but because they also produced the blocking factor (the antibodies) that prevents T cells from doing their rightful job (as the Hellströms discovered). Now the story is not so simple. Instead of just one way of destroying cancer cells (the T cell), the immune system is now known to have at least four different ways, and almost certainly there are more just waiting to be uncovered (Figure 24).

The technique T cells use to destroy cancer cells is very ingenious and the details are just being worked out. Anthony Allison and his colleagues at the Clinical Research Centre near London found during the middle of 1973 that T lymphocytes punch holes in cancer cell membranes by perverting a technique used in normal intercellular communication.

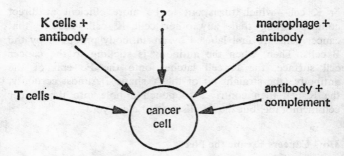

Figure 24. The four known ways in which the immune system can attack cancer cells. There may be more waiting to be discovered.

When normal cells approach each other they sometimes create tiny communication channels between each other by fusing a small part of their membranes together to form a microscopic intercellular tube. T cells do this with cancer cells, but as soon as the tube is made they break away after first making sure that the cancer cell cannot repair the small hole left in its membrane. The contents of the cancer cell begin to leak out, water pours in, until finally the cell bursts.

B cells have now shed their entirely negative image because immunologists have recently discovered that some antibodies, interacting with the complement system, can also severely damage cancer cells.

Macrophages can join in the battle against cancer too. They can kill cancer cells either non-specifically as they do any foreign material they find in the body, or specifically if they are armed with antibody complex which will direct them to specific cancer cells.

During 1972 and 1973 another type of cell has moved onto the anti-cancer scene. It looks like a lymphocyte, and has some characteristics of B cells, but it isn't. Researchers in America, Britain and Sweden discovered the cell—which toward the end of 1973 was officially named a killer cell,

or K cell—which turns out to be more efficient at direct
contact killing than any other cell. K cells require that
cancer cells are first labeled by an antibody produced by the
B cells. Then, when the antibody is sticking to the cancer
cell surface, the K cell latches onto the Fc end of the
antibody (the straight bit of the Y shape). Almost certainly,
the K cell then contrives to punch a hole into the cancer
cell membrane, but the details are not clear yet.

How Cancers Escape the Net

Thirty-nine out of forty incipient cancers are destroyed
before they become established. What concerns immunologists
is how the fortieth escapes.

BLOCKING FACTORS

The Hellströms, and the many others who followed their
example, have already demonstrated that there is some kind
of blocking factor in the blood of cancer patients preventing
active lymphocytes attacking the cancer cells. As soon as the
blocking factor came to light, there started a long—and
continuing—search to discover what it is. Initially the Hellströms thought the factor was anti-tumor antibody coating
the cancer cell preventing the T cells approaching (hence
the B cells' bad reputation, because they produce the antibody). But by 1971 the University of Washington researchers had concluded that the blocking factor was a
complex between tumor antigen and anti-tumor antibody.
Robert Baldwin of Nottingham University, England, also
has good evidence that blocking is caused by an antibody/
antigen complex. This complex could therefore bind to the
T cell (via the antigen part of the complex) or to the cancer
cell (via the antibody). Either way, T cell activity would
be thwarted.

Meanwhile researchers at the Chester Beatty Research
Institute in London had been enmeshed in the same problem.

In December 1972 one of them, Graham Currie, published a paper claiming that the blocking resulted simply from excess tumor antigen circulating in the blood and blocking the surface of potentially aggressive T cells. He had done tests on human patients with skin cancer in which he took out just a few of the cancer cells, inactivated them and then reinjected them back directly into one of the patient's lymph nodes. He found that this treatment boosted the patient's anti-cancer antibody production and allowed a significant, but transient, regression of the tumors. Currie claimed that the effect of the extra antibody was to mop up the cancer antigen flowing in the blood, thus allowing the T cells access to the cancer cells. But because the cancer cells are continually shedding masses of antigen into the blood, the previous blocking levels were soon reestablished.

Currie suggests that if the blocking factor is indeed solubilized cancer antigen, then one could explain how a tumor establishes itself in the first place. He says that a small developing cancer can release antigen in a limited locality, thus causing local blocking. There is good evidence for such local blocking: if a small tumor is transplanted from one area in an experimental animal to another in the same animal the tumor probably will be rejected. This shows that the tumor is immunogenic, but that in its original locality the immune response is blocked. As a small tumor grows, it releases more and more antigen, according to Currie, and its area of blocking influence spreads. When the whole body has blocking factor circulating around it, cells from the primary tumor can break off and establish outposts (known as metastases) elsewhere.

Arguments about the exact nature of the blocking factor continue. It may be that blocking is caused by free cancer antigen and antigen/antibody complexes. Again, the argument is not academic, because immunologists need to know exactly what the block is caused by so they can do something about it.

ENHANCEMENT

Immunologists have known since the late 1950s that if they inject anti-cancer antibody from one animal into another bearing the same kind of tumor there is a good chance that the tumor will grow better, rather than be destroyed. Tumor enhancement, as it is known, remained a mystery until the closing days of 1973.

During 1972 Richard Prehn of the Institute of Cancer Research in Philadelphia predicted that what might enhance tumor growth was a small specific immune response. And so it turned out. While a group of researchers at Washington University School of Medicine were tackling another problem of cancer cells, they stumbled across the answer to Prehn's prediction quite by accident. Eventually they confirmed that although high levels of specific anti-tumor antibody are able to destroy the cancer cell, low levels actually stimulate the tumor to greater growth. Exposed to low levels of antibody, cancer cells grow almost twenty times faster than normal.

Immunologists are discovering that many human tumors are weakly antigenic; that is, they possess foreign antigens, but the immune response provoked is only mild. In the light of these latest results, weak antigenicity not only helps tumors escape the lethal attentions of the immune system in the early stages of growth, it actually helps to boost the tumor's growth. When he was postulating that antibody might help tumor growth, Prehn concluded that it is a positive advantage for a tumor to be antigenic, as long as the response provoked is not too great. He said that "this would provide an explanation of the fact that most, and perhaps all, tumors are antigenic."

The researchers at Washington University School of Medicine—William Shearer, Gordon Philpott, and Charles Parker—suggest that the reason that cancer cells are stimulated by low levels of antibody might have something to do with the altered molecular patterning on the tumor cell surface.

The new patterns might form a growth trigger that is set off by interaction with antibody.

ANTIGEN MODULATION

One way of avoiding serious immunological attack while retaining the ability to be antigenically foreign if the occasion suits is by a process known as antigenic modulation. Edward Boyse and Lloyd Old, two scientists now working at the Memorial Sloan-Kettering Cancer Center, discovered this curious phenomenon in the late 1960s.

Boyse and Old found that when tumor cells are persistently exposed to moderate levels of antibody, specific antigens on the cell surface disappear. Remove the antibody and the antigens come back again. (A good analogy is a field of rabbits [the antigens] that jump down their burrows for cover when a man with a gun [the antibodies] comes along.) This fascinating cell surface behavior still remains something of an enigma. It may be simply a variant of normal cell behavior, or it could be specific to tumor cells. Immunologists do not know yet. Either way, antigenic modulation might easily help the cancer cells survive in a hostile environment.

SPECIFIC IMMUNOLOGICAL DEFICIENCY

As we said earlier, defective immune response genes might make an individual particularly vulnerable to some kind of immune challenge. If the immune deficiency involves an inability to react to cancer-causing organisms or to operate immunological surveillance efficiently, particular types of cancers would be able to flourish in that individual.

Immunological Intervention in Cancer

It is no exaggeration to claim that immunological techniques offer the best hope available for conquering cancer. It is also no exaggeration to say that such claims have been on the lips of immunologists for many years now, and that

desirable goal is still very much a thing of the future.
But with enormous strides made even just within the past
two years scientists can now see more clearly than ever
before the potential specific applications of immunology in
the fight against cancer. Possible clinical applications fall
within three groups: diagnosis, prophylaxis and therapy.

IMMUNODIAGNOSIS

One consequence of characterizing cancer antigens will
almost certainly be the development of new techniques for
diagnosing cancer at an early stage, and of monitoring the
disease during treatment.

The fact that tumors shed antigens which may or may not
combine with antibody to form blocking factors opens the
way to detecting new cancers and watching the progress of
established tumors. Clinicians know already that if a tumor-
bearing patient has only a small amount of blocking factor
in his blood the prognosis is good, whereas an abundance
of blocking factor implies that the tumor has a high chance
of resisting immunological attack. Diagnosing tumors before
other clinical symptoms appear depends of course on the cross-
reactivity of cancer antigens.

The fetal antigens that are sometimes associated with
tumors are already the basis of diagnostic tests, but there
are problems. For instance, carcinoembryonic antigen (CEA)
is almost always linked with cancer of the intestine, and the
antigen is produced early in the disease. This antigen was
first recognized in the mid-1960s. Since then immunologists
have realized that it is not exclusively associated with in-
testinal tumors. Other tumors sometimes release it, and some
people have detectable levels of the antigen in their blood
in the absence of a tumor. At the moment it seems that
CEA possibly has a better role in monitoring established
tumors than in diagnosing new ones.

A second fetal antigen that is catching the clinician's eye
is α-feto protein. This antigen was first discovered in associa-

tion with rat liver cancers in the early 1960s by Russian researchers. In 1964 a-feto protein was found in a human patient with liver cancer. Since then only one other type of cancer (teratoblastoma) has been associated with the antigen, and this is not very common. And a survey reported in 1970 that only two cases out of more than five thousand had no tumor when a-feto protein was detected. In other words, the rate of so-called false positives is very low.

Because liver cancer is often a fairly rapid disease, it can present problems for early diagnosis. For instance, a French scientist working at the International Agency for Cancer Research tells of a man in Africa in whom they got a positive result for a-feto protein. On surgical examination the doctors could find no signs of liver cancer at all. Six weeks later, the man died, of liver cancer.

In spite of these problems, immunodiagnosis promises to have an important impact on the crucial area of early detection of cancer.

IMMUNOPROPHYLAXIS

Now that so many diseases caused by microorganisms can be prevented by vaccination, the next step is to look for vaccination against cancer. This must be some way off yet for humans, but it is by no means a notion of pure fantasy.

What immunologists need in order to vaccinate effectively is a specific, important antigen to aim at. In domestic chickens this has already been done with Marek's disease. This is a tumor of the lymphoid system caused by a herpes virus (related to the one involved in Burkitt's lymphoma). In this case, the chickens are vaccinated against the virus, so that the organism itself and cells bearing viral antigens will be attacked. If a definite causal relationship between a virus and a human tumor could be established, prophylactic vaccination could be contemplated. Certainly, there are a number of cancer researchers who would like to try vaccination against the herpes virus associated with Burkitt's lymphoma. Another human tumor in which a viral cause is suspected,

therefore opening the way to some kind of vaccination, is
leukemia.

Virus-induced tumors are the best bets for prophylatic
vaccination, but if other human tumors proved to have
immunogenic cross-reacting antigens, the same approach
would be possible there too. As Graham Currie put it in 1973,
"The very existence of cross-reacting cell-membrane antigens
does at least provide a basis for optimism about the im-
munoprophylaxis of malignant disease."

IMMUNOTHERAPY

Surgery, chemotherapy and radiotherapy form the major
modes of attack on cancer at the moment. Because cancer
cells are undoubtedly foreign to the body (they are immunologically non-self), immunotherapy must very soon become
the fourth mode of attack against malignant disease, and
there is every chance that it will become *the* mode of attack.

Attempts at immunotherapy go back almost a hundred
years. Some of the earliest efforts—motivated more by the
feeling that there was nothing to lose rather than by a
rational approach—were fairly gruesome. Nevertheless,
some attempts succeeded simply because they managed to
nudge the immune systems into extra activity. Currently there
are two main approaches to immunotherapy: specific and
non-specific. In the former immunologists are trying to direct
the immune system's attack directly to specific cancer antigens. In the latter, the idea is to boost the activity of the
immune system overall in the hope that cancer cells will
succumb.

SPECIFIC IMMUNOTHERAPY

There are immunologists the world over attempting to
find ways of boosting the undoubted—but blocked—immune
response to tumors. Currie and his colleagues in London
showed in 1973 that by taking a sample of a patient's

tumor and reinjecting the cells into another part of the body it is possible to boost the specific immune response. Although in itself not a therapeutic technique, it does raise optimism for exploiting a patient's own defenses. Av Mitchison, London University, argues that there is no reason why one should not remove T cells from a cancer patient, clean them up to remove the blocking factor and then replace them in the patient. A combination of the two approaches might be quite effective.

A recurrent problem with cancers is the weak immunogenicity of their antigens. A number of researchers are trying to get round this by linking other antigenic determinants to the cancer antigens. For instance, George Klein in Sweden finds that if he vaccinates mice with influenza viruses cultured in tumor cells, the animals are able to raise a greater than usual immune response against that type of tumor. While they are growing in the tumor cells in the laboratory, some tumor antigens become linked with viral antigens. When the "hybrid" viruses are injected into the mice the immune response generates immunity both to the viral antigens and to some of the tumor antigens. The idea of vaccinating people with viruses that have been cultured in tumor cells is not acceptable as a prophylactic or therapeutic technique in humans. But encouraged by the success in mice, researchers are now looking for other techniques of linking tumor antigens to other helper determinants.

NON-SPECIFIC IMMUNOTHERAPY

Non-specific ways of boosting the immune response of a cancer patient had their beginnings at the end of the nineteenth century. In 1893 William Coley, an American surgeon, injected a mixture of bacterial products into a sixteen-year-old boy dying of cancer. Over a period of a few months the tumor shrank and finally disappeared. Coley tried this approach because he had noticed remarkable remissions in cancer patients who contracted simple bacterial infections.

After his success with the boy, Coley treated several hundred more people, many of whom clearly benefited. Unfortunately, Coley's work went unrecognized, but it has its parallel today with the use of the tuberculosis vaccine called BCG.

When it is injected into patients BCG generates anti-BCG antibodies. Researchers in America, France and Britain have now demonstrated convincingly that BCG treatment can destroy cancer cells too by boosting the patient's general immune responsiveness. For instance, Donald Morton at the University of California and Edmund Klein at Roswell Park Memorial Institute in Buffalo are using BCG on patients with skin cancer; Virginia Capse Livingston has achieved remissions in patients with breast cancer; Ray Powles and his colleagues at St. Bartholomew's Hospital in London are conducting encouraging tests during 1973 and 1974 on leukemia therapy; and Georges Mathé at the Paul Brousse Hospital near Paris has reported a number of successes with various forms of leukemia.

Mathé explains that the great benefit of immunotherapy of cancer is that, if it works, it destroys every last cancer cell, something that none of the other modes of treatment can do. And unlike chemotherapy and radiotherapy, immunotherapy does not destroy normal cells in the body; the only target is the tumor. In most of Mathé's trials he has combined immunotherapy with controlled chemotherapy: the attack is biphasic. The anti-cancer chemicals destroy the bulk of the tumor, and the immunotherapy completes the job.

TRANSFER FACTOR

One offbeat technique currently going through clinical trials to test its anti-cancer efficacy involves a mysterious substance known as transfer factor. Discovered more than twenty years ago by New York University researcher Sherwood Lawrence, transfer factor appears to be able to carry specific immunity from one set of lymphocytes to another. For example, if transfer factor is extracted from lymphocytes reacting to the tuberculosis organism, the factor can induce anti-tuberculosis activity in other lymphocytes with which it comes into contact—transfer factor appears to carry the immunological anti-tuberculosis message.

In spite of their long acquaintance with transfer factor, immunologists are still not sure about its chemical nature. Some think it is made of ribonucleic acid (RNA), the molecule that carries messages from the nucleus to the rest of the cell. Others believe it is RNA linked to a small protein molecule. The point about transfer factor, though, is that it works—doctors have successfully transferred immunity to specific pathogens to patients deficient in the required immune response.

The problem with treating cancer by transfer factor therapy is the difficulty in obtaining lymphocytes sensitized to specific cancers. Possible sources are relatives of cancer patients (with certain cancers, people in close contact with patients have marked anti-cancer immune responses) and cancer patients who have recovered from the disease. Once the specific transfer factor is isolated it can be used to treat the lymphocytes of a cancer patient; the treated lymphocytes will then have specific anti-cancer activity. Although there is a long way to go yet, preliminary results look encouraging. Transfer factor may prove to be the most specific method of all of boosting a cancer patient's anti-cancer immune response.

Any treatment of cancer faces the problem that if there is even one single cancer cell left at the end of the treatment there is a great danger that it will proliferate and establish the cancer once again. Immunotherapy will destroy that last cell, and this is why it is such a potentially valuable form of treatment. As we have seen, the number of ways our immune systems can attack cancer is now much greater than was thought even two years ago. This greater flexibility offers more subtle opportunities for manipulating the immune system to the benefit of cancer patients.

Transplants

If you must have an organ transplant you would be wise to ensure that you are an identical twin. If, like the vast majority of the population, you don't have a genetic copy of yourself walking the streets, the fate of your transplant depends on the skill of the doctors in preventing the organ from being rejected. For although the surgery involved in organ transplants can be very intricate, the success or failure of the operation depends largely on the immunological response to the graft.

A grafted organ is rejected because its specific histocompatibility antigens are recognized as being foreign by the recipient's immune system. Ever since organ transplantation really got under way in the early 1960s, the technique for overcoming this very specific response has been, metaphorically, to hit it with a sledge hammer. When a patient receives a new organ (from a donor who has been chosen as a close match of histocompatibility antigens so as to minimize the rejection problem) he will probably be put on a mixture of drugs, each of which helps to block an immune response. But the block is broad and undiscriminating—the whole immune response is damped down, thus putting the patient at risk from infections.

The drug mixture currently in favor includes azathioprine, prednisone with the occasional use of anti-lymphocyte globulin (ALG). The action of the first two is to stop cells growing and dividing. Because the immune response depends on a rapid expansion of specific cell populations, this general anti-growth activity hits the immune system hardest. ALG is usually an antibody against human lymphocytes produced by injecting lymphocytes into a horse. The anti-lymphocyte serum (ALS) can be purified to isolate the important globulin component (ALG). ALG attacks lymphocytes and therefore prevents an immune response. A combination of drugs is used because to give any one of them singly in a dose high enough to prevent an immune response would probably be toxic.

After receiving his new organ the patient will probably face a series of rejection crises in which rejection reaction begins to be mounted. With careful treatment, and a bit of luck, these crises can be overcome and the organ will eventually be accepted. Intensive immunosuppressive treatment can be maintained only for a few months. It can be stepped up to cope with rejection crises, but eventually drug treatment can be reduced to a low, monitoring level, but not stopped altogether. By some as yet unexplained means the patient eventually comes to tolerate the graft much more than in the initial post-operative stage. According to the Kidney Transplant Registry, current success rates for closely matched kidney transplants (living, related donors) is close to 80 per cent for two years. For grafts from cadavers, the figure is closer to 50 per cent. To improve these success rate substantially, new methods are clearly needed.

FUTURE METHODS OF IMMUNOSUPPRESSION

With increasing knowledge about the mechanisms of tolerance and the nature of the histocompatibility antigens, immunologists are now beginning to think in terms of more specific methods for easing an organ into a transplant patient. The two main techniques currently at the fore of these developments exploit the phenomena of enhancement and tolerance. If successful, these new methods of blocking a specific immune response will yield two main benefits: first, organ survival times will improve, eventually approaching 100 per cent success; second, the secondary hazards from drug toxicity and other infections that accompany current immunosuppressive therapy will be avoided.

Enhancement was discovered almost by accident in the early 1930s by American immunologist Nathan Kayliss. He discovered that if he injected tumor cells into an experimental animal, and then followed that immediately with antibodies specific to that tumor, the tumor would grow and flourish much more so than if no antibody was given. The phenomenon is explained partially in terms of blocking: the antibody binds to the surface of the tumor, but doesn't kill it; the layer of antibody on the tumor cell surface then prevents the lethal approaches of the anti-cancer T cells (and other aggressive cells) as is postulated for normal cancer growth.

Some immunologists have been arguing that enhancement might be exploited to protect organ grafts. In other words, an organ should be implanted into a patient, together with specific antibodies against the organ. The first clinical trial of this kind was performed at Guy's Hospital, London, in 1970. The recipient's kidney was provided by his mother, and the anti-donor serum by his father. Although the outcome was not dramatic, the kidney survived with rather less than normal immunosuppressive drug therapy being required. Since 1970 progress has been somewhat slow on this front, and the potential of the technique—considerable though it is—still remains to be proved.

The second technique, tolerance, is probably the most attractive of all. The idea of pre-treating a recipient with donor antigens, thus inducing specific tolerance to a subsequent graft, seems almost too good to be true, and perhaps it is. A number of researchers are currently examining the possibilities of inducing some degree of specific immunological unresponsiveness (another phrase for tolerance) in graft recipients; prominent among these is Leslie Brent and his colleagues at St. Mary's Hospital Medical School, London.

In the last couple of years Brent has developed a system for experimental animals with which he can induce permanent tolerance to a graft in between 30 and 40 per cent of rat recipients. He gives the recipient animals a single injection of liver extract (containing donor antigens) from the potential donors about twenty days before the tansplant operation. (He also gives the animals anti-lymphocytic serum— and a bacterial preparation, known as *Bacillus pertussis,* which potentiates the ALS—for a few days after the transplant.) The result of all this is to produce good organ survival rates, many of which are permanent.

With higher survival rates, this technique would seem to be the answer to the transplant surgeon's problems. But there are a number of practical difficulties. For instance, although it is easy to have access to specific donor cells some weeks before transplantation when using experimental animals, this is not the case with humans. The most convenient source of donor organs is cadavers. This means that organs to be transplanted would have to be stored for up to two weeks while tolerance is being induced in the potential recipient. At the moment there is no way of preserving human organs, like kidneys and hearts, for this length of time. Maybe someone will come up with one. Meanwhile Brent has suggested developing what he calls a "universal antigen cocktail" made up of a selection of all the important human histocompatibility antigens. A universal tolerance could then be induced in potential recipients.

Transplant immunology is clearly on the brink of a new era. The days of relying on sledge-hammer immunosuppression through drugs may soon be replaced by a more sophisticated immunosuppression through enhancement and tolerance. In a paper at the end of 1973 Frank Stuart of the Department of Surgery, University of Chicago, described the current situation as follows: "Since its beginnings, clinical kidney transplantation has progressed through a series of plateaus. It has been stalled for several years, but the prospects are bright that immunologically specific suppression of allograft rejection can be achieved within the decade. The door will then be open for transplantation of any organ or tissue for which surgical techniques are available."

We are all Transplants

It is appropriate to end this chapter, and the whole book, by reminding you that we all started life as a transplant: the fetus in its mother's uterus is in part antigenically foreign (those antigens from the father), and therefore ought to provoke an immune rejection response. Why developing fetuses escape this immunological fate is yet another mystery of immunology.

Research into this curious phenomenon has been slow to start, but it is now gathering pace. Obvious questions have been asked about the immunological relationship: Does the fetus sport transplantation antigens during its development? Is the amount of shared antigenicity between mother and fetus enough to allow the latter to be tolerated?

The answer to the first question is a very definite yes. Chemical tests show that by the time the fetus is a mere two cells big (that is, the ovum has divided once) it displays its antigens for all to see. Two experiments demonstrate that the answer to the second question (about shared antigens) is no. Tissues taken from a developing fetus and transplanted to another part of the mother's body are promptly rejected. And a fetus can be transplanted into the uterus of a genetically different "foster" mother without harm.

Another possibility once considered is that the uterus might be what is called an immunologically privileged site. The front chamber of the eye, and the brain are examples of such sites. These structures are not served by lymph vessels (a necessary condition if an immune response is to be initiated) and will therefore tolerate grafts. It is possible to create privileged sites experimentally, a trick developed by Clyde Barker of the University of Pennsylvania School of Medicine. He isolated a flap of skin on the back of a guinea pig, but left the blood vessels intact. This flap of skin, whose lymph vessels have been destroyed, can then be induced to tolerate foreign grafts for long periods, just like a fetus. This is a nice idea for the uterus, but the fact is that it is well served with lymph vessels, and it can be provoked into various types of immune response to prove the point.

One of the favorite ways of probing the mechanics of a mother's tolerance of her fetus is to transplant other tissues into the uterus to see if it is possible to induce her to tolerate these too. The idea behind it is to determine whether the uterus acts as some kind of protective barrier for the potential offspring. Alan Beer and Rupert Billingham of the University of Texas Health Center at Dallas have pursued this technique extensively and they are forced to conclude that, as a protective barrier, the uterus is pretty poor. It *is* possible to get a tissue graft to be tolerated for longer than usual inside a uterus, particularly if the experimental animal has the sex hormones estrogen and progesterone pumped into it to simulate pregnancy. The uterus must therefore afford some degree of protection because grafts elsewhere on such a "pseudo-pregnant" animal are rejected almost as quickly as normal, and certainly faster than in the uterus. But the uterus does not provide the whole answer.

The main protection of the fetus must therefore come from somewhere other than the uterus—probably the fetus (and accompanying tissues) itself. The fetus, which is wrapped snugly inside a fluid-filled sac, is linked to the wall of the uterus via the placenta, a large structure looking not unlike a red jellyfish. The placenta, which carries fetal blood, is in very intimate contact with the uterine wall, so much so that food and oxygen can pass from maternal blood into the fetal blood; the two blood systems do not actually mix. Although the bloods do not mix in the formal sense, there is a very small drift of blood cells (red and white) from mother to fetus and vice versa.

In a series of clever cross-matching experiments in rats, Beer and Billingham have shown that maternal lymphocytes can pass readily into the fetus and under certain circumstances damage it, causing a short-lived runt to be born. Their latest experiments lead the Texas researchers to believe that under normal conditions any anti-fetal lymphocytes are inactivated by blocking antibody, just as some cancers are protected against immunological attack. They conclude this because they find that it is possible to immunize a female animal against her own fetus, provided the immunization is done so that when the fetus is vulnerable, the mother's antibody response has not yet been mounted fully. In these circumstances the mother does inflict immunological damage on her offspring. But when this female has a second litter, no harm is done—the antibody level has built up and the cell-mediated anti-graft attack is prevented by the blocking antibody.

It appears that even if some lymphocytes do get through to the fetus, they are likely to meet at least a small defensive response. Arthur Silverstone of John Hopkins School of Medicine finds that when sheep fetuses are about halfway through their gestation they are capable of at least a limited immunological response—they can reject skin grafts, for instance. Maternal lymphocytes (which may or may not be blocked with antibody) which happen to stray into the fetus are therefore likely to be mopped up pretty swiftly. Indeed, maternal lymphocytes may well be the first foreign invader that the offspring's immune defenses have to repel.

Probably the most important factor in fetal protection, however, comes from the placenta, or rather the thin layer of cells that actually come into contact with the uterus wall. This layer of cells, known as the trophoblast, appears to be non-antigenic—it can be transplanted to various parts of a foreign host without provoking an immunological reaction. The invulnerability of the trophoblast may lie in the so-called glycocalyx, a chemical coating on top of the cells which may mask the antigens; this coat may also repel approaching lymphocytes.

Clearly, there are a number of separate factors shielding the developing fetus from immunological attack. But, whatever are the mechanisms, it is nice to know that our mothers tolerate us before we are born, if not after!

Bibliography

Immunology is such a fast-moving science that few textbooks can hope to be abreast of current ideas. Readers can refer back to a number of standard texts to go more deeply into historical ideas, but for more detail of the up-to-date ideas in this book annual volumes and periodicals are the best source.

For background on the evolution of the immune system, on early ideas of immunology and cancer and of aging, plus a general view of clonal selection:

Immunological Surveillance
  by Frank Macfarlane Burnet
  Pergamon Press, 1970
  and

The Immunological Theory of Aging
  by Roy Walford
  Munksgaard 1969

FOR REVIEWS OF CURRENT IDEAS:

Clinical Immunobiology
  ed. by Fritz Bach and Robert Good
  Academic Press
  the first volume was published in 1973

FOR REPORTS OF CURRENT WORK:

Science—a weekly academic journal
Scientific American—a monthly magazine
New Scientist—a weekly popular science magazine

INDEX

2292